Optavia Diet Cookbook

200 Juicy, And Easy To Make Recipes For Your Long Term Transformation. Start Your Rapid Weight Loss Journey Trough These Healthy Low-Carb Recipes On a Budget

Sophie Haye

Sophie Haye

© Copyright 2021 - All rights reserved.

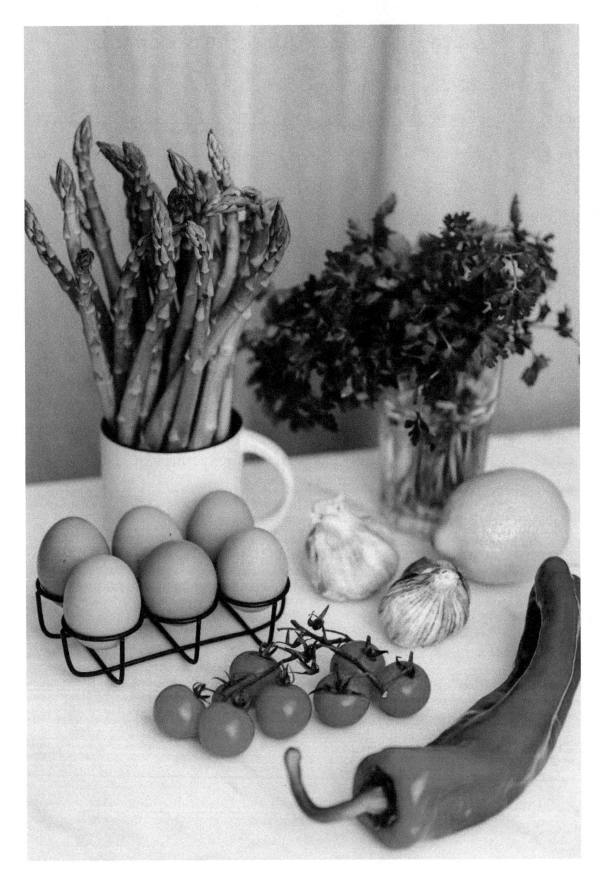

Table Of Contents

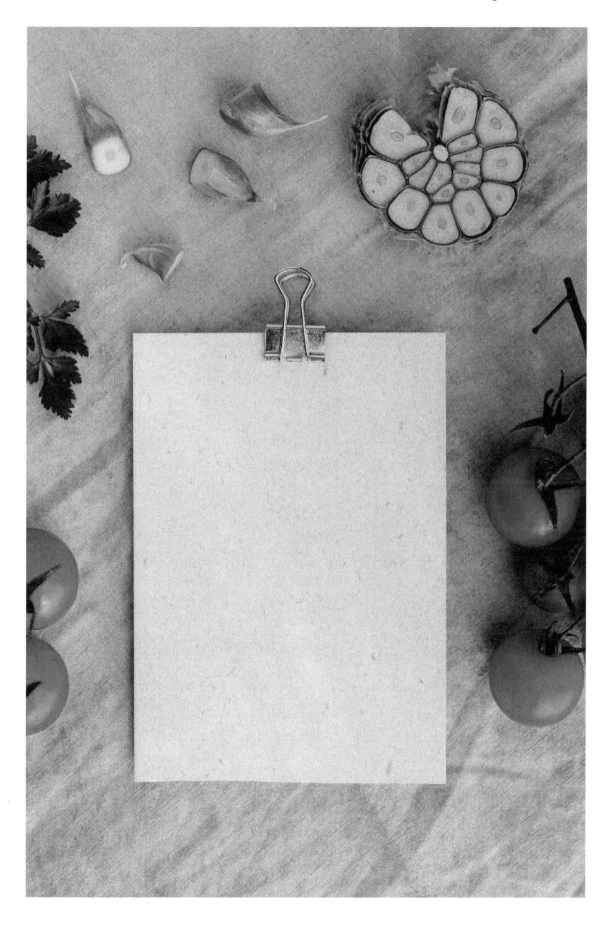

Introduction

This Optavia Diet Cookbook is intended to help people lose fat and weight by the reduction of carbohydrates and calories. The mayor benefits of weight loss and limited sodium utilization are the reduced risk of heart disease (through reduction in blood pressure) and type 2 diabetes.

The following 200 Recipes are:

- high-protein based - as protein serves as a carb alternative when the body needs energy
- made off ingredients that can be easily found at discount grocery
- characterized by simple and stress-free instructions that require no cooking experience.

There's no excuse not to cook healthy!

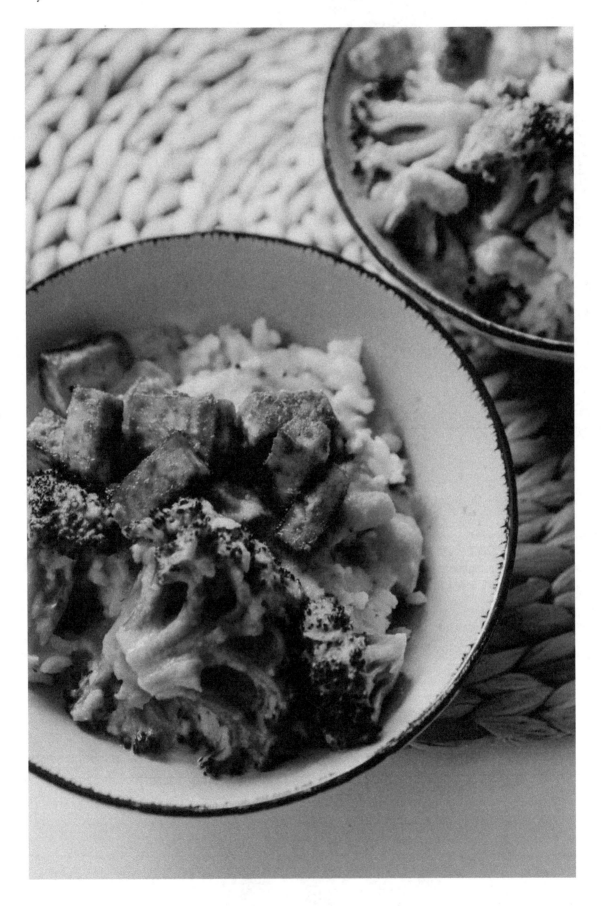

Chapter 1:

Foods To Eat And Avoid

Benefits of Optavia Diet

Why is this Lean and Green strategy so effective? There are few key reasons:

1) Less Carbs – The vast majority of us eat far too many carbs in general, so our insulin levels are constantly elevated. Insulin is a storage hormone that whisks excess glucose out of our bloodstream into fat cells (assuming our glucose storage tanks – our muscles and liver – are full). Insulin is released when we eat carbohydrates, especially starchy, sugary, and processed carbohydrates. By limiting carbohydrate intake at night, we are in effect controlling the insulin our bodies release.

2) Veggies are "free" food – Vegetables are the perfect food for fat loss because eating them is like "free" food. What I mean is that the amount of calories a vegetable contains is usually burned off during digestion. So it's really like you're eating food that provides no calories. In fact, some vegetables like lettuce require your digestive system to burn more calories than the lettuce contains! This concept is known as negative calorie balance. To top it off, veggies contain ample amounts of fiber, which help you feel more satiated. Needless to say, if you are trying to lose fat, veggies should be an important part of your nutrition strategy.

Lean and Green Fast Fat Loss 4

3) Less Calories – The overall calories you consume in a day are usually less when you cut out starchy carbs at night. Most people have their largest (and unhealthiest) meal at dinner, right before going to bed. This may not be a good idea because eating too much right before you go to sleep can affect quality of your sleep and is associated with weight gain. If you go Lean and Green, then you are looking at 300-500 calories depending on how much healthy fat you have and how much meat you consume. That's a solid range.

This type of strategy is also used by natural bodybuilders and fitness models, but it's known as "carbohydrate tapering". The idea is that our bodies are best able to utilize carbohydrates for energy in the beginning of the day, so as the day wears on, less carbs should be consumed to allow for maximum fat burning. In addition, most carbs that people eat are generally the empty calorie variety. I'm not suggesting you have to cut carbs at night in order to lose fat and that all carbs are bad. In fact, I prefer a moderate carb diet to a low carb diet. While low carb diets have been proven by mountains of research to lead to faster fat loss, they're also notoriously difficult to maintain (there's the catch!). So people who go "on" low carb diets inevitably gain the weight back when they go "off" the diet. That's why the Lean and Green is a "nutrition strategy", something to have in your bag of tricks.

What Can I Eat?

All Recipes listed in this cookbook contains these foods:

1. Healthy Fats , such as avocado, flaxseed, walnut, or olive oil;

2. Greens and Non-Starchy Vegetables, divided into higher, moderate, and lower carbohydrate categories such as:

    - Higher Carb: Peppers or Broccoli

    - Moderate Carb: Summer squash or Cauliflower

    - Lower Carb: Salad greens

3. Lean Meats, classified in

    - Lean: Pork chops, lamb, or salmon

    - Leaner: Chicken breast or swordfish

    - Leanest: Egg whites, shrimp, and cod

What Can I Not Eat?

For healthier eating habits, it's advisable to avoid use of:

1. Alcohol

2. Sugary Beverages, as energy drinks, juice, or soda

3. High-Calorie Additions , as High-fat salad dressings, shortening and butter

4. Indulgent Desserts, such as ice cream, cookies, or cakes

Chapter 2:

Lean and Green Risotto and Pasta

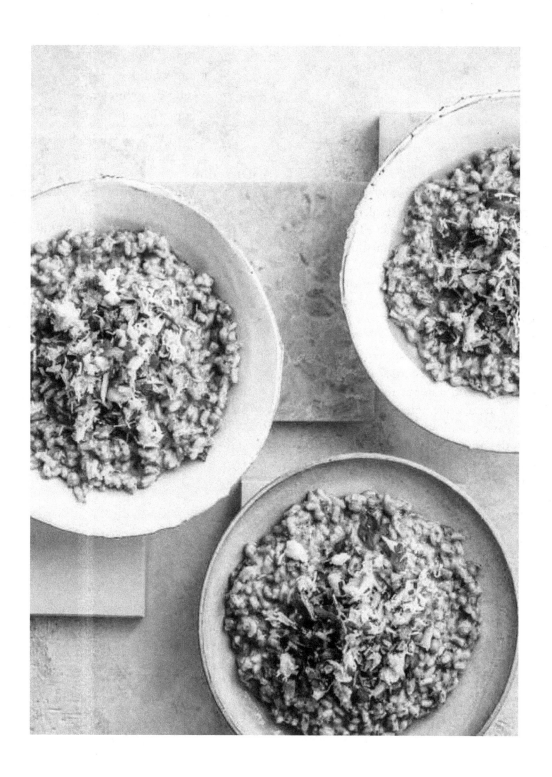

Cauliflower Asparagus Risotto with Chicken

Preparation Time: 5 minutes
Cooking Time: 25 minutes
Servings: 4
Ingredients:

- 4 tablespoons. of large flake nutritional yeast
- ½ cup chicken stock
- ¼ pound asparagus should be chopped
- 1 ¼ pound grated or riced cauliflower
- 2 tablespoons butter, to be melted
- ¼ teaspoon each pepper and salt
- 2 pounds boneless, skinless chicken breasts.

Directions:

1. Preheat the oven to over 350°F.
2. Place the chicken in a casserole dish, then season with pepper and salt. Then pour the already melted butter in the chicken and roast until the chicken's internal temperature reaches 165°F in about 30 minutes. Remove from the oven and place aside.
3. In your pot, combine asparagus, cauliflower rice, and chicken stock and simmer it until it becomes tender. You just need to add water as required.
4. When you are done, remove the asparagus risotto and cauliflower from the stove and stir in the nutritional yeast. Then serve the risotto together with the roasted chicken breast.

Nutritional value:
Calories: 320 kcal
Protein: 43g
Carbohydrate: 13 g
Fat: 11 g

Fennel Wild Rice Risotto

Preparation Time: 5 minutes
Cooking Time: 35 minutes
Servings: 6
Ingredients:

- 2 tablespoons extra virgin olive oil
- 1 shallot, chopped
- 2 garlic cloves, minced
- 1 fennel bulb, chopped
- 1 cup wild rice
- ¼ cup dry white wine
- 2 cups chicken stock
- 1 teaspoon grated orange zest
- Salt and pepper to taste

Directions:

1. Heat the oil in a heavy saucepan.
2. Add the garlic, shallot and fennel and cook for a few minutes until softened.
3. Stir in the rice and cook for 2 additional minutes then add the wine, stock and orange zest, with salt and pepper to taste.
4. Cook on low heat for 20 minutes.
5. Serve the risotto warm and fresh.

Nutritional value:
Calories: 162 kcal
Fat: 2 g
Protein: 8 g
Carbohydrates: 20 g

Barley Risotto

Preparation Time: 15 minutes
Cooking Time: 7 to 8 hours
Servings: 8
Ingredients:

- 2¼ cups hulled barley, rinsed
- 1 onion, finely chopped
- 4 garlic cloves, minced
- 8 ounces button mushrooms, chopped
- 6 cups low-sodium vegetable broth
- ½ teaspoon dried marjoram leaves
- ⅛ teaspoon freshly ground black pepper
- ⅔ cup grated parmesan cheese

Directions:

1. In a 6-quart slow cooker, mix the barley, onion, garlic, mushrooms, broth, marjoram, and pepper.
2. Cover and cook on low heat for 7 to 8 hours, or until the barley has absorbed most of the liquid and is tender, and the vegetables are tender.
3. Stir in the Parmesan cheese and serve.

Nutritional value:
Calories: 288 kcal
Carbohydrates: 45 g
Sugar: 2 g
Fiber: 9 g
Fat: 6 g
Saturated Fat: 3 g
Protein: 13 g
Sodium: 495 mg

Risotto with Green Beans, Sweet Potatoes, and Peas

Preparation Time: 20 minutes
Cooking Time: 4 to 5 hours
Servings: 8
Ingredients:

- 1 large sweet potato, peeled and chopped
- 1 onion, chopped
- 5 garlic cloves, minced
- 2 cups short-grain brown rice
- 1 teaspoon dried thyme leaves
- 7 cups low-sodium vegetable broth
- 2 cups green beans, cut in half crosswise
- 2 cups frozen baby peas
- 3 tablespoons unsalted butter
- 1/2 cup grated Parmesan cheese

Directions:

1. In a 6-quart slow cooker, mix the sweet potato, onion, garlic, rice, thyme, and broth.
2. Cover and cook on low heat for 3 to 4 hours, or until the rice is tender.
3. Stir in the green beans and frozen peas.
4. Put the lid on and cook on low for 30 to 40 minutes or until the vegetables are tender.
5. Stir in the butter and cheese. Put the lid on and cook on low heat for 20 minutes, then stir and serve.

Nutritional value:
Calories: 385 kcal
Carbohydrates: 52 g
Sugar: 4 g Fiber: 6 g
Fat: 10 g Saturated Fat: 5 g
Protein: 10 g Sodium: 426 mg

Shrimp and Tomato Linguini
Preparation Time: 10 minutes
Cooking Time: 20 minutes
Servings: 6
Ingredients:

- 1 ounce extra-virgin olive oil
- 3 minced cloves garlic
- 32 ounces tomatoes, diced
- 8 ounces dry white wine
- 1 ounce butter
- A pinch salt and black pepper
- 16 ounces uncooked linguine pasta
- 16 ounces medium shrimp, peeled and deveined
- 1 teaspoon Cajun seasoning
- 1 ounce extra-virgin olive oil

Directions:

1. Heat 1 ounce of olive oil in a large stock pot on Medium Heat
2. Sauté garlic in the oil for 2 minutes, then add tomatoes and wine to the garlic and oil
3. Cook the mixture for 30 minutes, stirring frequently, then add butter, salt and pepper
4. Boil a large pot of salted water and cook the linguine for 10-12 minutes or until al dente
5. Drain water from the pool and set noodles aside
6. Sprinkle shrimp with seasoning, salt and pepper and cook in a frying pan with 1 ounce of olive oil on Medium heat.
7. Stir for 5 minutes or until pink in the center.
8. Add shrimp to the pasta sauce, then toss with the linguine in a large bowl and serve

Nutritional value:
Fats: 10.7 g Cholesterol: 4 g
Sodium: 98.2 mg Potassium: 135.1 mg
Carbohydrates: 3.8 g

Creamy Penne
Preparation Time: 10 minutes
Cooking Time: 25 minutes
Servings: 4
Ingredients:

- ½ cup penne, dried
- 9 ounces chicken fillet
- 1 teaspoon Italian seasoning
- 1 tablespoon olive oil
- 1 tomato, chopped
- 1 cup heavy cream
- 1 tablespoon fresh basil, chopped
- ½ teaspoon salt
- 2 ounces Parmesan, grated
- 1 cup water, for cooking

Directions:

1. Pour water in the pan, add penne, and boil it for 15 minutes. Then drain water.
2. Pour olive oil in the skillet and heat it up.
3. Slice the chicken fillet and put it in the hot oil.
4. Sprinkle the chicken with the Italian seasoning and roast for 2 minutes each side.
5. Then add fresh basil, salt, tomato, and grated cheese.
6. Stir well.
7. Add heavy cream and cooked penne.
8. Cook the meal for 5 minutes more over the medium heat. Stir it from time to time.

Nutritional value:
Calories 388 kcal
Fat 23.4 g Fiber 0.2 g
Carbs 17.6 g Protein 17.6 g

Chapter 3:

Lean and Green Soup Recipes

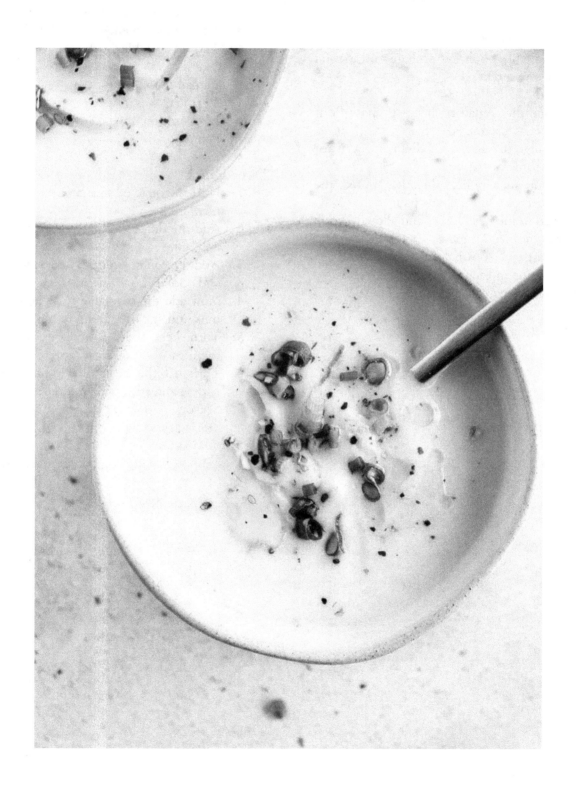

Sophie Haye

Tomato Basil Soup
Preparation Time: 5 minutes
Cooking Time: 10 minutes
Servings: 2
Ingredients:

- 1 cup tomatoes, chopped
- ½ cup of water
- 1 cup basil leaves
- One tablespoon low-sodium and low-fat cheese, shredded

Directions:

1. Place the tomatoes in a saucepan. Pour water. Close the lid.
2. Change the heat to medium and wait for the tomatoes to boil.
3. Using a handheld blender, puree the tomatoes while still in a pan.
4. Add in the basil leaves and allow to cook for another 2 minutes.
5. Scoop in bowls and serve with ½ tablespoon each of shredded cheese.

Nutritional value:
Calories per serving: 137 kcal
Protein: 1.7g
Carbs: 3g
Fat: 0.9g
Sugar: 0.9g

Creamy Cauliflower Soup
Preparation Time: 15 minutes
Cooking Time: 15 minutes
Servings: 6
Ingredients:

- 5 cups cauliflower rice
- 8 ounces cheddar cheese, grated
- 2 cups unsweetened almond milk
- 2 cups vegetable stock
- 2 tablespoon water
- 1 small onion, chopped
- 2 garlic cloves, minced
- 1 tablespoon olive oil
- Pepper
- Salt

Directions:

1. Heat the olive oil in a large stockpot over medium heat.
2. Add the onion and garlic and cook for 1-2 minutes.
3. Add the cauliflower rice and water. Cover and cook for 5-7 minutes.
4. Now add the vegetable stock and almond milk and stir well. Bring to boil.
5. Turn heat to low and simmer for 5 minutes.
6. Turn off the heat. Slowly add cheddar cheese and stir until smooth.
7. Season soup with pepper and salt.
8. Stir well and serve hot.

Nutritional value:
Calories: 214 kcal Fat: 15 g Carbs: 3 g Sugar: 3 g
Protein: 16 g Cholesterol: 40 mg

Chicken Breast Soup

Preparation Time: 5 minutes
Cooking Time: 4 hours
Servings: 4
Ingredients:

- 3 chicken breasts, skinless, boneless, cubed
- 2 celery stalks, chopped
- 2 carrots, chopped
- 2 tablespoons olive oil
- 1 red onion, chopped
- 3 garlic cloves, minced
- 4 cups chicken stock
- 1 tablespoon parsley, chopped

Directions:

1. In your slow cooker, mix all the ingredients except for the parsley, cover and cook on high heat for 4 hours.
2. Add the parsley, stir, ladle the soup into bowls and serve.

Nutritional value: Calories 445 kcal Fat 21.1 g Fiber 1.6 g Carbs 7.4 g Protein 54.3 g

Cheeseburger Soup

Preparation Time: 20 minutes
Cooking Time: 25 minutes
Servings: 4
Ingredients:

- ¼ cup of chopped onion
- 1 can (14.5 ounces) diced tomato
- 1 pound of 90% lean ground beef
- ¾ cup of diced celery
- 2 teaspoon of Worcestershire sauce
- 3 cups of low sodium chicken broth
- ¼ teaspoon of salt
- 1 teaspoon of dried parsley
- 7 cups of baby spinach
- ¼ teaspoon of ground pepper
- 4 ounces of reduced-fat shredded cheddar cheese

Directions:

1. Get a large soup pot and cook the beef until it becomes brown. Add the celery, onion, and sauté until it becomes tender. Remove from the fire and drain excess liquid.
2. Stir in the broth, tomatoes, parsley, Worcestershire sauce, pepper, and salt. Cover and allow it to simmer on low–heat for about 20 minutes
3. Add spinach and leave it to cook until it becomes wilted in about 1–3 minutes. Top each of your servings with 1 ounce of cheese.

Nutritional value:
Calories: 400 kcal
Carbohydrate: 11 g
Protein: 44 g
Fat: 20 g

Chapter 4:

Lean and Green Salmon Recipes

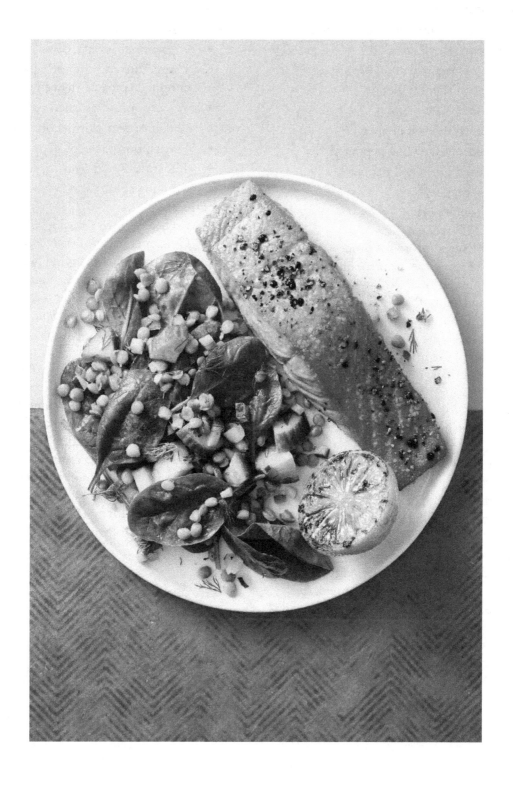

Savory Cilantro Salmon
Preparation Time: 10 minutes
Cooking Time: 30 minutes
Servings: 4
Ingredients:

- 2 tablespoons of fresh lime or lemon
- 4 cups of fresh cilantro, divided
- 2 tablespoon of hot red pepper sauce
- ½ teaspoon of salt, divided
- 1 teaspoon of cumin
- 4.7 unces. of salmon filets
- ½ cup water
- 2 cups sliced red bell pepper
- 2 cups sliced yellow bell pepper
- 2 cups sliced green bell pepper
- Cooking spray
- ½ teaspoon pepper

Directions:

1. Get a blender or food processor and combine half of the cilantro, limejuice or lemon, cumin, hot red pepper sauce, water, and salt; then puree until they become smooth. Transfer the marinade gotten into a large re-sealable plastic bag.
2. Add salmon to marinade. Seal the bag, squeeze out air that might have been trapped inside, turn to coat salmon. Refrigerate for about 1 hour, turning as often as possible.
3. Now, after marinating, preheat the oven to about 400°F. Arrange the pepper slices in a single layer in a slightly greased, medium-sized square baking dish. Bake it for 20 minutes and turn the pepper slices once.
4. Drain your salmon and do away with the marinade. Crust the upper part of the salmon with the remaining chopped, fresh cilantro. Place salmon on the top of the pepper slices and bake for about 12–14 minutes until you observe that the fish flakes easily when it is being tested with a fork. Enjoy.

Nutritional value:
Calories: 350 kcal, Carbohydrate: 15 g
Protein: 42 g, Fat: 13 g

Salmon Florentine
Preparation Time: 5 minutes
Cooking Time: 30 minutes
Servings: 4
Ingredients:

- 1 ½ cups of chopped cherry tomatoes
- ½ cup of chopped green onions
- 2 garlic cloves, minced
- 1 teaspoon of olive oil
- 1 quantity of 12 oz. package frozen chopped spinach, thawed and patted dry
- ¼ teaspoon of crushed red pepper flakes
- ½ cup of part-skim ricotta cheese
- ¼ teaspoon each for pepper and salt
- 4 quantities of 5 ½ oz. wild salmon fillets
- Cooking spray

Directions:

1. Preheat the oven to 350°F
2. Get a medium skillet to cook onions in oil until they start to soften, which should be in about 2 minutes. You can then add garlic inside the skillet and cook for an extra minute. Add the spinach, red pepper flakes, tomatoes, pepper, and salt. Cook for 2 minutes while stirring. Remove the pan from the heat and let it cool for about 10 minutes. Stir in the ricotta.
3. Put a quarter of the spinach mixture on top of each salmon fillet. Place the fillets on a slightly greased rimmed baking sheet and bake it for 15 minutes or until you are sure that the salmon has been thoroughly cooked.

Nutritional value: Calories: 350 kcal Carbohydrate: 15 g Protein: 42 g Fat: 13 g

Wild Salmon

Preparation Time: 15 minutes
Cooking Time: 35 minutes **Servings:** 4
Ingredients:

- 4 or 6 ounce farmed salmon.
- 2 teaspoons butter.
- Smashed garlic.
- 1 tablespoon salt to taste
- 1 tablespoon dried basil leaves
- 4 wedge or raw lemons

Directions:

1. Stir the basil, garlic powder and salt together in a bowl.
2. Then rub them on the salmon fillets equally.
3. Over medium heat, melt the butter.
4. Cook the salmon in the butter until it turns brown on each side.
5. Serve the salmon together with a lemon wedge.

Nutritional value:

Calories: 390.4 kcal

Fats: 27.7 g	Cholesterol: 82.5 mg
Sodium: 356.1 mg	Carbohydrates: 3.6 g
Dietary Fiber: 0.8 g	Protein: 32.0 g

Baked Mustard Salmon

Preparation Time: 20 minutes
Cooking Time: 15 minutes
Servings: 2
Ingredients:

- 2 salmon fillets
- 1 tablespoon mustard paste
- ½ teaspoon chili paste
- ½ teaspoon garlic powder
- ½ teaspoon ginger powder
- 1 pinch salt
- 1 pinch cayenne pepper
- 1 tablespoon olive oil

Directions:

1. Marinate the salmon using mustard, chili paste, garlic, ginger, salt, cayenne, and let it sit for 20 minutes.
2. Preheat the oven to 390°F.
3. Place aluminum foil on your baking sheet.
4. Add the fish on the baking sheet.
5. Add olive oil on top. Bake for 8 minutes.
6. Flip them carefully and bake for 7 minutes.
7. Serve.

Nutritional value:

Fat: 5.1 g

Cholesterol: 82.6 mg

Sodium: 286.5 mg

Potassium 498.5 mg

Carbohydrate: 5.0 g

Foil Packet Salmon

Preparation Time: 5 minutes
Cooking Time: 15 minutes
Servings: 2
Ingredients:

- 2 x 4 ounces salmon fillets, skinless
- 2 tablespoon unsalted butter, melted
- ½ teaspoon garlic powder
- 1 lemon, medium sized
- ½ teaspoon dried dill

Directions:

1. Take a sheet of aluminum foil and cut into two squares measuring about 5" x 5". Lay each of the salmon fillets at the center of each piece. Brush both fillets with a tablespoon of butter and season it with a quarter-teaspoon of garlic powder.
2. Halve the lemon and grate the skin of one of the pieces over the fish. Cut the lemon in four slices, using two to top each fillet. Season each fillet with a quarter-teaspoon of dill.
3. Fold the tops and sides of the aluminum foil over the fish to create a kind of package. Place each one in the fryer.
4. Cook for twelve minutes at 400°F.
5. The salmon is ready when it flakes easily.
6. Serve hot.

Nutritional value:

Calories: 240 kcal   Fat: 13g
Protein: 21g   Sugar: 9g

Salmon Patties

Preparation Time: 10 minutes
Cooking Time: 7 minutes
Servings: 2
Ingredients:

- 8 ounces salmon fillet, minced
- 1 lemon, sliced
- ½ teaspoon garlic powder
- 1 egg, lightly beaten
- ⅛ teaspoon salt

Directions:

1. Add all the ingredients, except the lemon slices, into the bowl and mix until well combined.
2. Spray the air fryer basket with cooking spray.
3. Place lemon slices into the air fryer basket.
4. Make an equal shape of patties from the salmon mixture and place them on top of the lemon slices into the air fryer basket.
5. Cook at 390°F for 7 minutes.
6. Serve and enjoy.

Nutritional value:

Calories: 184 kcal   Fat: 9.2 g
Carbohydrates: 1 g   Sugar: 0.4 g
Protein: 24.9 g
Cholesterol: 132 mg

Perfect Salmon Fillets

Preparation Time: 10 minutes
Cooking Time: 15 minutes
Servings: 2
Ingredients:

- 2 salmon fillets
- 1/2 teaspoon garlic powder
- 1/4 cup plain yogurt
- 1 teaspoon fresh lemon juice
- 1 tablespoon fresh dill, chopped
- 1 lemon, sliced
- Pepper
- Salt

Directions:

1. Place the lemon slices into the air fryer basket.
2. Season the salmon with pepper and salt and place it on top of the lemon slices and into the air fryer basket.
3. Cook salmon at 330°F for 15 minutes.
4. Meanwhile, in a bowl, mix together the yogurt, garlic powder, lemon juice, dill, pepper, and salt.
5. Place the salmon on a plate and top with the yogurt mixture.
6. Serve and enjoy.

Nutritional value: Calories: 195 kcal Fat: 7 g Carbohydrates: 6 g Sugar: 2 g Protein: 24 g Cholesterol: 65 mg

Nutritious Salmon

Preparation Time: 10 minutes
Cooking Time: 10 minutes
Servings: 2
Ingredients:

1. 2 salmon fillets
2. 1 tablespoon olive oil
3. ¼ teaspoon ground cardamom
4. ½ teaspoon paprika
5. Salt

Directions:

1. Preheat the air fryer to 350°F.
2. Coat the salmon fillets with olive oil and season with paprika, cardamom, and salt and place it into the air fryer basket.
3. Cook the salmon for 10-12 minutes. Turn them halfway through.
4. Serve and enjoy.

Nutritional value:

Calories: 160 kcal Fat: 1 g
Carbohydrates: 1 g
Sugar: 0.5 g Protein: 22 g
Cholesterol: 60 mg

Sophie Haye

Lemon Chili Salmon
Preparation Time: 10 minutes
Cooking Time: 17 minutes
Servings: 4
Ingredients:
- 2 pounds salmon fillet, skinless and boneless
- 2 lemon, juiced
- 1 orange, juiced
- 1 tablespoon olive oil
- 1 pinch fresh dill
- 1 chili, sliced
- Pepper
- Salt

Directions:
1. Preheat the air fryer to 325 °F.
2. Place the salmon fillets in the air fryer baking pan and drizzle with the olive oil, lemon juice, and orange juice.
3. Sprinkle chili slices over the salmon and season it with pepper and salt.
4. Place the pan in the air fryer and cook for 15-17 minutes.
5. Decorate with dill and serve.

Nutritional value:
Calories: 339 kcal   Fat: 17.5 g Carbohydrates: 2
Sugar: 2 g Protein: 44 g   Cholesterol:
100 mg

Curry Salmon with Mustard
Preparation Time: 10 minutes
Cooking Time: 8 minutes
Servings: 4
Ingredients:
¼ teaspoon ground red pepper or chili powder
¼ teaspoon ground turmeric
¼ teaspoon salt
1 teaspoon honey
1/8 teaspoon garlic powder or a minced clove garlic
2 teaspoons. whole grain mustard
4 pcs 6-oz salmon fillets

Directions:
1. In a small bowl mix well salt, garlic powder, red pepper, turmeric, honey and mustard.
2. Preheat oven to broil and grease a baking dish with cooking spray.
3. Place salmon on baking dish with skin side down and spread evenly mustard mixture on top of salmon.
4. Pop in the oven and broil until flaky around 8 minutes.

Nutritional value:
Calories: 324 kcal
Fat: 18.9 g Protein: 34 g
Carbs: 2.9 g

Chapter 5:

Other Lean and Green Fish Recipes

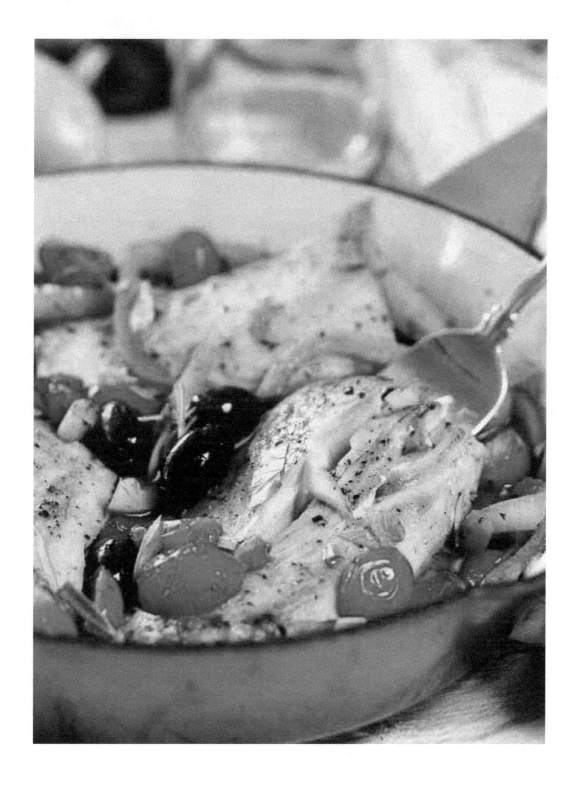

Baked Cod & Vegetables

Preparation Time: 15 minutes
Cooking Time: 15 minutes
Servings: 4
Ingredients:

- 1 pound cod fillets
- 8 ounces asparagus, chopped
- 3 cups broccoli, chopped
- ¼ cup parsley, minced
- ½ teaspoon lemon pepper seasoning
- ½ teaspoon paprika
- ¼ cup olive oil
- ¼ cup lemon juice
- 1 teaspoon salt

Directions:

1. Preheat the oven to 400°F. Cover a baking sheet with parchment paper and set aside.
2. In a small bowl, combine the lemon juice, paprika, olive oil, pepper spices, and salt.
3. Place the fish fillets in the center of the greaseproof paper. Arrange the broccoli and asparagus around the fish fillets.
4. Pour lemon juice mixture over the fish fillets and top with parsley.
5. Bake in a preheated oven for 13-15 minutes.
6. Serve and enjoy.

Nutritional value:
Calories: 240 kcal
Fat: 11g   Carbs: 6 g
Sugar: 6 g   Protein: 27 g
Cholesterol: 56 mg

Steamed White Fish Street Tacos

Preparation Time: 5 minutes
Cooking Time: 25 minutes
Servings: 8
Ingredients:

- 6 ounces avocado, sliced
- 6 large romaine lettuce leaves
- 1 tablespoon lime juice
- 2 tablespoons chopped fresh cilantro
- ½ cup diced tomato
- ½ teaspoon salt, to be divided
- ½ teaspoon garlic powder
- 1-pound raw cod filets

Directions:

1. Season the cod with ¼ teaspoon of salt and garlic powder. Steam the fish until it is thoroughly cooked, which should take about 5-10 minutes. Peel the fish, using either a fork or your fingers, remove all the bones.
2. Meanwhile, get a small bowl and prepare pico de gallo. Combine the red onion, cilantro, jalapeno, lime juice, tomato, and the remaining ¼ teaspoon of salt.
3. To prepare the tacos, top each of the romaine lettuce leaves with avocado, fish, and pico de gallo.

Nutritional value:
Calories: 360 kcal
 Protein: 44g
Carbohydrate: 15 g
Fat: 14 g

Pan Fried Catfish

Preparation Time: 10 minutes
Cooking Time: 30 minutes
Servings: 6
Ingredients:

- 1 cup Cornmeal
- 2 teaspoon paprika
- 2 teaspoon ground cayenne pepper
- 4 Catfish fillets (4 ounces)
- 1 teaspoon onion powder
- 1/3 cup Extra virgin olive oil
- 1 cup milk
- Garlic (4 cloves).

Directions:

1. Using a mixing bowl, stir the cayenne pepper, onion powder, and paprika together with the cornmeal.
2. Proceed to mix it thoroughly, and then pour the mixture into a waxed paper sheet.
3. Heat your oil in a large pan using medium heat.
4. Pour the milk into a bowl and dip the catfish fillets into the milk, ensure you hold the fillets up so the milk can drip off.
5. Next, get your cornmeal mixture and roll the fillet soaked with milk in it.
6. Completely cover the fillet with the cornmeal mixture before setting it aside.
7. Put your garlic clove into the heated oil and fry, ensure you do not burn it.
8. Next, add the catfish fillets covered with cornmeal and cover to cook for about 6-7 minutes, turning to the sides while it fries.
9. Do not forget to sprinkle salt while turning the fish.
10. Cook until it is golden brown, and then drain on paper towels.

Note: To allow for even distribution of oil over the fish's surface, coat the fillets lightly instead of the pan.

Nutritional value:
Fats: 11 g
Cholesterol: 75 mg
Sodium: 490 mg
Carbohydrates: 16 g   Protein: 23 g

Seafood Paella

Preparation Time: 5 minutes
Cooking Time: 45 minutes
Servings: 8
Ingredients:

- 2 tablespoons extra virgin olive oil
- 1 shallot, chopped
- 2 garlic cloves, chopped
- 1 red bell pepper, cored and diced
- 1 carrot, diced
- 2 tomatoes, peeled and diced
- 1 cup wild rice
- 1 cup tomato juice
- 2 cups chicken stock
- 1 chicken breast, cubed
- Salt and pepper to taste
- 2 monkfish fillets, cubed
- ½ pound fresh shrimps, peeled and deveined
- ½ pound prawns
- 1 thyme sprig
- 1 rosemary sprig

Directions:

1. Heat the oil in a skillet and stir in the shallot, garlic, bell pepper, carrot and tomatoes. Cook for a few minutes until softened.
2. Stir in the rice, tomato juice, stock, chicken, salt and pepper and cook on low heat for 20 minutes.
3. Add the rest of the ingredients and cook for 10 additional minutes.
4. Serve the paella warm and fresh.

Nutritional value:
Calories: 245 kcal
Fat: 8 g
Protein: 27 g
Carbohydrates: 20.6 g

Lemon Dill Trout

Preparation Time: 10 minutes
Cooking Time: 10 minutes
Servings: 1
Ingredients:

- 2 pounds pan-dressed trout (or other small fish)
- 1 ½ teaspoon salt
- ½ cup butter or margarine
- 2 tablespoons McCormick's Dill Weed
- 3 tablespoons lemon juice

Directions:

1. Cut the fish lengthwise and season it with the salt.
2. Prepare a frying pan by melting the butter with the McCormick's Dill Weed.
3. Fry the fish on a high heat, flesh side down, for 2-3 minutes per side.
4. Remove the fish. Add the lemon juice to the butter and Dill Weed to create a sauce.
5. Serve the fish with the sauce.

Nutritional value:
Calories: 367 kcal
Carbs: 25 g
Fat: 14 g
Protein: 40 g
Fiber: 21 g

Sesame Tuna Steak

Preparation Time: 5 minutes
Cooking Time: 12 minutes
Servings: 2
Ingredients:

- 1 tablespoon coconut oil, melted
- 2 x 6 ounces tuna steaks
- ½ teaspoon garlic powder
- 2 teaspoon black sesame seeds
- 2 teaspoon white sesame seeds

Directions:

1. Apply the coconut oil to the tuna steaks with a brush, then season it with garlic powder.
2. Combine the black and white sesame seeds. Embed them in the tuna steaks, covering all the fish. Place the tuna into your air fryer.
3. Cook for eight minutes at 400°F, turn the fish at the 4 minutes mark.
4. The tuna steaks are ready when they have reached a temperature of 145°F.
5. Serve straightaway.

Nutritional value:
Calories: 160 kcal
Fat: 6g
Protein: 26g
Sugar: 7g

Lemon Garlic Shrimp

Preparation Time: 10 minutes
Cooking Time: 15 minutes
Servings: 2
Ingredients:

- 1 lemon, medium sized
- ½ pounds medium shrimp, shelled and deveined
- ½ teaspoon Old Bay seasoning
- 2 tablespoon unsalted butter, melted
- ½ teaspoon minced garlic

Directions:

1. Grate the rind of the lemon into a bowl. Cut the lemon in half and juice it in the same bowl. Toss in the shrimp, Old Bay seasoning, and butter, mix everything and make sure the shrimp is completely covered.
2. Transfer to a round baking dish about six inches wide, then place the dish in your fryer.
3. Cook at 400°F for six minutes. The shrimp is cooked when it turns a bright pink color.
4. Serve hot, drizzle any leftover sauce over the shrimp.

Nutritional value:

Calories: 490 kcal

Fat: 9g

Protein: 12g

Sugar: 11g

Foil Packet Lobster Tail

Preparation Time: 5 minutes
Cooking Time: 15 minutes
Servings: 2
Ingredients:

- 2 x 6 ounces lobster tail halves
- 2 tablespoon salted butter, melted
- ½ medium lemon, juiced
- ½ teaspoon Old Bay seasoning
- 1 teaspoon dried parsley

Directions:

1. Lay each lobster on a sheet of aluminum foil. Pour a light drizzle of melted butter and lemon juice over each one, and season with Old Bay.
2. Fold down the sides and ends of the foil to seal the lobster. Place each one in the fryer.
3. Cook at 375°F for twelve minutes.
4. Just before serving, top the lobster with dried parsley.

Nutritional value:

Calories: 510 kcal

Fat: 18g Protein: 26g

Sugar: 12g

Lemon Butter Scallops

Preparation Time: 15 minutes
Cooking Time: 30 minutes
Servings: 1
Ingredients:

- 1 lemon
- 1 pound scallops
- ½ cup butter
- ¼ cup parsley, chopped

Directions:

1. Juice the lemon into a Ziploc bag.
2. Wash your scallops, dry them, and season to taste. Put them in the bag with the lemon juice. Refrigerate for an hour.
3. Remove the bag from the refrigerator and leave for about twenty minutes until it returns to room temperature. Transfer the scallops into a foil pan that is small enough to be placed inside the fryer.
4. Preheat the fryer at 400°F and put the rack inside.
5. Place the foil pan on the rack and cook for five minutes.
6. In the meantime, melt the butter in a saucepan over a medium heat. Zest the lemon over the saucepan, then add in the chopped parsley. Mix well.
7. Be careful when removing the pan from the fryer. Transfer the contents to a plate and drizzle with the lemon-butter mixture.
8. Serve hot.

Nutritional value:
Calories: 420 kcal
Fat: 12g
Protein: 23g
Sugar: 13g

Cheesy Lemon Halibut

Preparation Time: 10 minutes
Cooking Time: 20 minutes
Servings: 2
Ingredients:

- 1 pound halibut fillet
- ½ cup butter
- 2 ½ tablespoon mayonnaise
- 2 ½ tablespoon lemon juice
- ¾ cup parmesan cheese, grated

Directions:

1. Preheat your fryer at 375°F.
2. Spray the halibut fillets with cooking spray and season as desired.
3. Put the halibut in the fryer and cook for twelve minutes.
4. In the meantime, mix the butter, mayonnaise, and lemon juice in a bowl with a hand mixer. Until a creamy texture is achieved.
5. Stir in the grated parmesan.
6. When the halibut is ready, open the drawer and spread the butter over the fish with a butter knife. Allow to cook for 2 more minutes, then serve hot.

Nutritional value:
Calories: 432 kcal Fat: 18g
Protein: 14g Sugar: 12g

Thyme Scallops

Preparation Time: 5 minutes
Cooking Time: 12 minutes
Servings: 1
Ingredients:
- 1 pounds scallops
- Salt and pepper
- ½ tablespoon butter
- ½ cup thyme, chopped

Directions:
1. Wash the scallops and dry them completely. Season with pepper and salt, then set aside while you prepare the pan.
2. Grease a foil pan in several spots with the butter and cover the bottom with the thyme. Place the scallops on top.
3. Preheat the fryer at 400°F and set the rack inside.
4. Place the foil pan on the rack and allow it to cook for seven minutes.
5. Be careful when removing the pan from the fryer and transfer the scallops to a serving dish.
6. Put any remaining butter in the pan over the fish and enjoy.

Nutritional value:
Calories: 291Cal Fat: 9g Protein: 17g
Sugar: 5g

Filipino Bistek

Preparation Time: 5 minutes
Cooking Time: 10 minutes
Servings: 4
Ingredients:
- 2 milkfish bellies, deboned and sliced into 4 portions
- ¾ teaspoon salt
- ¼ teaspoon ground black pepper
- ¼ teaspoon cumin powder
- 2 tablespoon calamansi juice
- 2 lemongrasses, trimmed and cut crosswise into small pieces
- ½ cup tamari sauce
- 2 tablespoon fish sauce
- 2 tablespoon sugar
- 1 teaspoon garlic powder
- ½ cup chicken broth
- 2 tablespoon olive oil

Directions:
1. Dry the fish using some paper towels.
2. Put the fish in a large bowl and coat with the rest of the ingredients. Allow it to marinate for 3 hours in the refrigerator.
3. Cook the fish steaks on an Air Fryer at 340°F for 5 minutes.
4. Turn the steaks over and allow them to grill for an additional 4 minutes. Cook until medium brown.
5. Serve with steamed white rice.

Nutritional value:
Calories: 259 kcal Fat: 3g Protein: 10g
Sugar: 2g

Sophie Haye

Saltine Fish Fillets
Preparation Time: 10 minutes
Cooking Time: 15 minutes
Servings: 4
Ingredients:
- 1 cup crushed saltines
- ¼ cup extra-virgin olive oil
- 1 teaspoon garlic powder
- ½ teaspoon shallot powder
- 1 egg, well whisked
- 4 white fish fillets
- Salt and ground black pepper to taste
- Fresh Italian parsley to serve

Directions:
1. In a shallow bowl, combine the crushed saltines and olive oil.
2. In a separate bowl, mix together the garlic powder, shallot powder, and the beaten egg.
3. Sprinkle a good amount of salt and pepper over the fish, before dipping each fillet into the egg mixture.
4. Coat the fillets with the crumb mixture.
5. Air fry the fish at 370°F for 10 - 12 minutes.
6. Serve with fresh parsley.

Nutritional value:
Calories: 502 kcal
Fat: 4g
Protein: 11g
Sugar: 9g

Dijon Mustard and Lime Marinated Shrimp
Preparation Time: 10 minutes
Cooking Time: 10 minutes
Servings: 8
Ingredients:
- ½ cup fresh lime juice, and lime zest as garnish
- ½ cup rice vinegar
- ½ teaspoon hot sauce
- 1 bay leaf
- 1 cup water
- 1 lb. uncooked shrimp, peeled and deveined
- 1 medium red onion, chopped
- 2 tablespoon capers
- 2 tablespoon Dijon mustard
- 3 whole cloves

Directions:
1. Mix hot sauce, mustard, capers, lime juice and onion in a shallow baking dish and set aside.
2. Bring to a boil in a large saucepan bay leaf, cloves, vinegar and water.
3. Once boiling, add shrimps and cook for a minute while stirring continuously.
4. Drain shrimps and pour shrimps into onion mixture.
5. For an hour, refrigerate while covered the shrimps.
6. Then serve shrimps cold and garnished with lime zest.

Nutritional value:
Calories: 232.2 kcal
Protein: 17.8g
Fat: 3g
Carbs: 15g

Dill Relish on White Sea Bass

Preparation Time: 10 minutes
Cooking Time: 12 minutes
Servings: 4
Ingredients:

- 1 ½ tablespoon chopped white onion
- 1 ½ teaspoon chopped fresh dill
- 1 lemon, quartered
- 1 teaspoon Dijon mustard
- 1 teaspoon lemon juice
- 1 teaspoon pickled baby capers, drained
- 4 pieces of 4-oz white sea bass fillets

Directions:

1. Preheat oven to 375oF.
2. Mix lemon juice, mustard, dill, capers and onions in a small bowl.
3. Prepare four aluminum foil squares and place 1 fillet per foil.
4. Squeeze a lemon wedge per fish.
5. Evenly divide into 4 the dill spread and drizzle over fillet.
6. Close the foil over the fish securely and pop in the oven.
7. Bake for 12 minutes or until fish is cooked through.
8. Remove from foil and transfer to a serving platter, serve and enjoy.

Nutritional value:

Calories: 115 kcal Protein: 7g Fat: 1g Carbs: 12g

Firecracker Shrimp

Preparation Time: 5 minutes
Cooking Time: 20 minutes **Servings:** 1
Ingredients:

- 11.2 ounces peeled shrimp
- 1 teaspoon lite soy sauce
- 2 teaspoon Walden Farms Apricot Preserves
- ½ teaspoon Sriracha sauce
- 1 teaspoon Sesame oil
- Also Needed: Soaked wooden or metal skewer

Directions:

1. Prepare the sauce by adding the apricot preserves into a microwavable dish and cooking until it's partially melted (20 seconds). Add the oil, soy sauce, and sriracha sauce to the melted apricot preserves; stirring until combined.
2. Thread the shrimp on the skewer.
3. Marinate the shrimp in the sauce for about an hour before grilling. If you are short of time, you can also brush the sauce over the shrimp before and during the grilling process.
4. Grill the shrimp with the lid off—using the medium temperature setting for two to three minutes per side.

Nutritional value:

Calories: 95 kcal
Protein: 1.59 g
Fat: 5.61 g
Carbohydrates: 10.29 g

Sophie Haye

Shrimp with Veggie

Preparation Time: 10 minutes
Cooking Time: 20 minutes
Servings: 4
Ingredients:

- 50 small shrimp
- 1 tablespoon Cajun seasoning
- 1 bag of frozen mix vegetables
- 1 tablespoon olive oil

Directions:

1. Cover the air fryer basket with aluminum foil.
2. Add all the ingredients into the large mixing bowl and mix it well.
3. Transfer shrimp and vegetable mixture into the air fryer basket and cook at 350°F for 10 minutes.
4. Toss well and cook for 10 more minutes..
5. Serve and enjoy.

Nutritional value:
Calories: 101 kcal
Fat: 4 g
Carbohydrates: 14 g
Sugar: 1 g
Protei:n 2 g
Cholesterol: 3 mg

Shrimp Scampi

Preparation Time: 10 minutes
Cooking Time: 10 minutes
Servings: 4
Ingredients:

- 1 pounds shrimp, peeled and deveined
- 10 garlic cloves, peeled
- 2 tablespoon olive oil
- 1 fresh lemon, cut into wedges
- ¼ cup parmesan cheese, grated
- 2 tablespoon butter, melted

Directions:

1. Preheat the air fryer to 370 °F.
2. Mix together the shrimp, lemon wedges, olive oil, and garlic cloves in a bowl.
3. Pour the shrimp mixture into the air fryer pan and place it into the air fryer and cook for 10 minutes.
4. Drizzle with melted butter and sprinkle with parmesan cheese.
5. Serve and enjoy.

Nutritional value:
Calories: 295 kcal
Fat: 17 g
Carbohydrates: 4 g   Sugar: 0.1 g
Protein: 29 g
Cholesterol: 260 mg

Seafood & Scallions Creole
Preparation Time: 10 minutes
Cooking Time: 30 minutes **Servings:** 5
Ingredients

- 4 tablespoons butter
- 1 large onion, diced
- 1 rib celery, diced
- 1 green bell pepper, diced
- 2 cloves garlic, minced
- ½ teaspoon salt
- ½ teaspoon thyme
- ½teaspoon black pepper
- ½ teaspoon cayenne pepper
- 1 tablespoon flour
- ⅓ cup dry white wine (optional)
- 15 ounces can of diced tomatoes, or about 1 ¼ cups fresh tomatoes, peeled and diced
- 1 cup chicken stock
- 2 bay leaves
- Hot pepper sauce, such as Tabasco, to taste
- 2 pounds large uncooked shrimp
- 6-8 cups hot cooked rice, for serving
- 2 green onions, chopped, for decorating

Directions:
1. In a large saucepan, heat 2 tablespoons of the butter over medium-high heat. Add the onion, celery, bell pepper, and garlic and cook, stirring, until softened, for about 3 minutes.
2. Add the shrimp and cook, stirring, until they turn pink, for about 2 minutes. Add in the salt, thyme, black pepper, and cayenne.
3. Add in the remaining 2 tablespoons of butter and melt it. Add in the flour and cook, stirring, for 1 minute, until it is cooked.
4. Add in the wine, tomatoes, stock, bay leaves, and hot pepper sauce. Reduce the heat to medium low and let it simmer, stirring occasionally, for 15 minutes.
5. Remove bay leaves. Using the back of a spoon, push the shrimp mixture to one side of the pot. Pour the eggs into the opposite side, and begin to scramble. Stir the eggs into the shrimp mixture and again push to one side. Pour the rice into the pot and mix it in. Cover the pot, reduce the heat to low, and cook for 5 more minutes until it's cooked through.
6. Sprinkle with green onions when serving

Nutritional value: Calories: 1017 kcal Protein: 89.27 g Fat: 52.71 g Carbohydrates: 95.46 g Calcium: 322 mg Magnesium: 1400 mg Phosphorus: 3672 mg

Garlic Shrimp & Broccoli
Preparation Time: 15 minutes and 30 minutes marinade **Cooking Time:** 8 minutes **Servings:** 4
Ingredients:

- ½ cup honey - ¼ cup soy sauce
- 1 teaspoon fresh grated ginger
- 2 tablespoons minced garlic
- ¼ teaspoon red pepper flakes
- ½ teaspoon cornstarch
- 1 pound large shrimp, peeled, deveined and tails removed if desired
- 2 tablespoon butter
- 2 cups chopped broccoli
- 1 teaspoon olive oil
- Salt and pepper

Directions:
1. In a large bowl, combine the honey, soy sauce, ginger, garlic, red pepper flakes, and cornstarch. Add shrimp and whisk to combine. Cover and refrigerate for 20 to 30 minutes.
2. In a large nonstick skillet, heat 1 tablespoon of the butter and olive oil over medium-high heat.
3. Cook and stir broccoli in a hot skillet until crisp-tender, stirring occasionally, for 2 to 4 minutes. Remove broccoli from the skillet.
4. Add the shrimp mixture to the hot skillet and stir-fry for 4-5 minutes or until the shrimps are done. Stir in the broccoli and add salt and pepper to taste.
5. Remove from the heat.
6. Serve with rice.

Nutritional value: Calories: 334 kcal rotein: 17.84 g Fat: 11.07 g Carbohydrates: 43.4 g Calcium: 100 mg Magnesium: 42 mg Phosphorus: 324 mg

Sophie Haye

Garlic Shrimp Zucchini Noodles
Preparation Time: 5 minutes
Cooking Time: 4 minutes
Servings: 5
Ingredients:

- 16 ounces uncooked shrimps, shelled and deveined
- One tablespoon olive oil
- 1 cup cherry tomatoes, cut in half
- 8 cups zucchini strips
- 2 tablespoons minced garlic
- 1 teaspoon dried oregano
- ½ teaspoon chili powder
- ½ teaspoon salt

Directions:

1. Brush the shrimps with olive oil. Place on a skillet and cook for 2 minutes on all sides or until pink. Set aside.
2. Place the rest of the fixings in a bowl and add the shrimps. Season with salt, then toss to coat the ingredients.

Nutritional value:
Calories per serving: 142 kcal
Protein: 19.7g
Carbs: 6.3g
Fat: 4.2g
Sugar: 3.8g

Italian Shrimp and Broccoli
Preparation Time: 20 minutes
Cooking Time: 20 minutes
Servings: 6
Ingredients:

- 7 ounces of fully cooked but frozen shrimp
- 1 cup of raw broccoli
- 1 tablespoon shredded Parmesan cheese
- ½ teaspoon of freshly ground black pepper
- 1 teaspoon of Olive oil
- ½ cup of chopped tomatoes
- 2 tablespoon of Ken's Lite Northern Italian to serve as dressing.

Directions:

1. Begin by defrosting the frozen shrimp.
2. Heat the olive oil and gradually add broccoli and tomatoes to it and leave for about 2-3 minutes.
3. Remove the skillet from heat, place the lid to cover and set it aside.
4. Scoop your dressing into another pan on fire, add your shrimp freshly ground pepper and fry until the shrimp turns opaque.
5. Place the shrimp and vegetables in one skillet/pan and cook for about 2-3 minutes extra.
6. Add the Parmesan cheese and then stir. Italian shrimp and broccoli are ready for consumption.

Nutritional value:
Fats: 12 g
Sodium: 830 mg
Carbohydrates: 34 g
Fibers: 3 g
Sugars: 4 g
Protein: 22 g

Mesquite Grilled Shrimp
Preparation Time: 15 minutes
Cooking Time: 10 minutes
Servings: 4
Ingredients:
- Seven ounces Big shrimps
- ¾ cup sliced courgettes
- ¾ cup Summer squash
- 1 Tablespoon seasoning with mesquite
- 1 tablespoon of olive oil
- Oregano (if wanted)

Directions:
1. Put oil on the grill.
2. Cover the courgettes and squash over the grill and sprinkle with the oregano.
3. Put 1 tablespoon of olive oil on the shrimp and sprinkle with mesquite seasoning.

Nutritional value:
Carbohydrates: 5 g
Protein: 35 g Fat: 14 g
Cholesterol: 459 mg
Sodium: 1991 mg
Potassium: 246 mg

Light Tuna Casserole
Preparation Time: 10 minutes
Cooking Time: 1 hour **Servings:** 6
Ingredients:
- 1 Cup of almond unsweetened milk
- 4 Low fat wedges Laughing cow garlic and herb cheese
- 1 cup low fat cheddar shredded cheese
- 1 Spoonful chives
- ¼ cayenne pepper in teaspoon
- 15–ounce drained tuna packed in water
- 2 Cups spaghetti cooked squash
- Salt & chilli to taste

Directions:
1. To make sauce: heat the almond milk, add the cheeses and stir until sauce thickens and melt.
2. Add the rest of ingredients to sprinkle on top reserving some of the cheddar cheese.
3. Spread over a casserole dish, sprinkle the cheese on top and bake at 350°F or until nice and hot for 30 minutes.
4. Depends on what you can eat, serves 2 to 4!
5. (Based on two servings, each serving is: slightly less than 1 lean, depends on the size of the tuna, 1 healthy fat, 2 greens and 1 ½ condiment)

Nutritional value:
Carbohydrates: 34.3g
Protein: 27.3g
Fat: 7 g,
Cholesterol: 34 mg
Sodium: 660 mg
Fiber: 3.6 g

Shrimp Skewers

Preparation Time: 10 minutes
Cooking Time: 5 minutes
Servings: 4
Ingredients:

- 1 cup medium shrimp, cleaned
- 1 teaspoon lemon juice
- 1 tablespoon Greek yogurt
- 1 pinch turmeric
- Salt and pepper to taste
- 1 teaspoons red chili powder
- 1 tablespoon almond butter

Directions:

1. Coat the shrimp in Greek yogurt, salt, pepper, red chili powder, lemon juice, and turmeric.
2. Let it sit for 10 minutes.
3. Thread them into wooden skewers.
4. In a pan, melt the butter.
5. Add the skewers on cook for 2 minutes per side.
6. Serve.

Nutritional value:
Fat: 1 g
Cholesterol 80 mg
Sodium 430 mg
Carbohydrate 0 g
Protein 11 g
Potassium 105 mg

Avocado Lime Shrimp Salad

Preparation Time: 15 minutes
Cooking Time: 0 minutes
Servings: 2
Ingredients:

- 14 ounces jumbo cooked shrimp, peeled and deveined; chopped
- 4 ½ ounces avocado, diced
- 1 ½ cup tomato, diced
- ¼ cup chopped green onion
- ¼ cup jalapeno with the seeds removed, diced fine
- 1 teaspoon olive oil
- 2 tablespoons lime juice
- ⅛ teaspoon salt
- 1 tablespoon chopped cilantro

Directions:

1. Get a small bowl and combine the green onion, olive oil, lime juice, pepper, a pinch of salt. Wait for about 5 minutes for all of them to marinate and mellow the flavor of the onion.
2. Get another large bowl and combined chopped shrimp, tomato, avocado, jalapeno. Combine all of the ingredients, add cilantro, and gently toss.
3. Add pepper and salt as desired.

Nutritional value:
Calories: 314 kcal   Protein: 26 g
Carbs: 15 g   Fiber: 9 g

Avocado Shrimp

Preparation Time: 10 minutes
Cooking Time: 20 minutes **Servings:** 2
Ingredients:

- ½ cup onion, chopped
- 2 pounds shrimp
- 1 tablespoon seasoned salt
- 1 avocado - ½ cup pecans, chopped

Directions:

1. Preheat the fryer at 400°F.
2. Put the chopped onion in the fryer and spray with some cooking spray. Leave to cook for five minutes.
3. Add the shrimp and set the timer for five minutes. Sprinkle some seasoned salt, then allow it to cook for five more minutes.
4. During these last five minutes, halve your avocado and remove the pit. Cut each half, then remove the flesh.
5. Be careful when removing the shrimp from the fryer. Place it on a dish and top with the avocado and the chopped pecans.

Nutritional value:

Calories: 195 kcal Fat: 14g

Protein: 36g Sugar: 10g

Avocado, Citrus, And Shrimp Salad

Preparation Time: 5 minutes **Cooking Time:** 4 minutes **Servings:** 4
Ingredients:

- 1 head green leaf lettuce
- 1 avocado
- ½ pound wild-caught shrimp
- 2 tablespoons olive oil
- Juice of 1 lemon

Directions:

1. Put the lettuce in a dish, then top with the mashed avocado.
2. Clean the shrimps by deveining and removing the head.
3. Heat the oil in a skillet using medium-low heat and heat the oil. Cook the shrimps for 2 minutes on each side.
4. Place the shrimps on top of the mashed avocado and drizzle with lemon juice.

Nutritional value:

Calories per serving: 359 kcal

Protein: 10.6g

Carbs: 50.1g

Fat: 7.5g

Sugar: 2.8g

Wild Rice Prawn Salad
Preparation Time: 5 minutes
Cooking Time: 35 minutes
Servings: 6
Ingredients:

- ¾ cup wild rice
- 1¾ cups chicken stock
- 1 pound prawns
- Salt and pepper to taste
- 2 tablespoons lemon juiced
- 2 tablespoons extra virgin olive oil
- 2 cups arugula

Directions:

1. Combine the rice and chicken stock in a saucepan and cook until the liquid has been absorbed entirely.
2. Transfer the rice to a salad bowl.
3. Season the prawns with salt and pepper and drizzle them with lemon juice and oil.
4. Heat a grill pan over medium flame.
5. Place the prawns on the hot pan and cook on each side for 2–3 minutes.
6. For the salad, combine the rice with arugula and prawns and mix well.
7. Serve the salad fresh.

Nutritional value:

Calories: 207 kcal   Fat: 4 g
Protein: 20.6 g   Carbohydrates: 17 g

Spicy Mackerel
Preparation Time: 10 minutes
Cooking Time: 20 minutes
Servings: 2
Ingredients:

- 2 mackerel fillets
- 2 tablespoon red chili flakes
- 2 teaspoon garlic, minced
- 1 teaspoon lemon juice

Directions:

1. Season the mackerel fillets with the red pepper flakes, minced garlic, and a drizzle of lemon juice. Allow to sit for five minutes.
2. Preheat your fryer at 350°F.
3. Cook the mackerel for five minutes, open the lid and flip the fillets, and allow them to cook on the other side for five more minutes.
4. Plate the fillets, and make sure to put any remaining juice over them before serving.

Nutritional value:

Calories: 240 Cal

Fat: 4g

Protein: 16g

Sugar: 3g

Crispy Calamari
Preparation Time: 5 minutes
Cooking Time: 15 minutes
Servings: 4
Ingredients:
- 1 pound fresh squid
- Salt and pepper
- 2 cups flour - 1 cup water
- 2 cloves garlic, minced
- ½ cup mayonnaise

Directions:
1. Remove the skin from the squid and discard any ink. Slice the squid into rings and season it with some salt and pepper.
2. Put the flour and water in separate bowls. Dip the squid first in the flour, then into the water, then into the flour again, ensuring that it is entirely covered with flour.
3. Preheat the fryer at 400°F. Put the squid inside and cook for six minutes.
4. In the meantime, prepare the aioli by combining the garlic with the mayonnaise in a bowl.
5. Once the squid is ready, plate up and serve with the aioli.

Nutritional value:

Calories: 247 kcal	Fat: 3g
Protein: 18g	Sugar: 3g

Air Fried Cod with Basil Vinaigrette
Preparation Time: 5 minutes
Cooking Time: 15 minutes
Servings: 4
Ingredients:
- ¼ cup olive oil
- 4 cod fillets
- A bunch of basil
- Juice from 1 lemon, freshly squeezed
- Salt and pepper to taste

Directions:
1. Preheat the air fryer for 5 minutes.
2. Season the cod fillets with salt and pepper to taste.
3. Place it in the air fryer and cook for 15 minutes at 3500°F.
4. Meanwhile, mix the rest of the ingredients in a bowl and whisk to combine.
5. Serve the air fried cod with the basil vinaigrette.

Nutritional value:
Calories 235 kcal Carbohydrates: 1.9g
Protein: 14.3g Fat: 18.9g

Grilled Mahi Mahi with Jicama Slaw

Preparation Time: 20 minutes **Cooking Time:**
10 minutes **Servings:** 4
Ingredients:

- 1 teaspoon each for pepper and salt, divided - 1 tablespoon lime juice, divided
- 2 tablespoon + 2 teaspoons of extra virgin olive oil
- 4 raw mahi-mahi fillets, which should be about 8 ounces each
- ½ cucumber which should be thinly cut into long strips like matchsticks (it should yield about 1 cup)
- 1 jicama, which should be thinly cut into long strips like matchsticks (it should yield about 3 cups) - 1 cup alfalfa sprouts - 2 cups coarsely chopped watercress

Directions:

1. Combine ½ teaspoon of both pepper and salt, 1 teaspoon of lime juice, and 2 teaspoons of oil in a small bowl. Then brush the mahi-mahi fillets all through with the olive oil mixture. Grill the mahi-mahi on medium-high heat until it becomes done (about 5 minutes,) turn it to the other side, and let it be done (about 5 minutes) (You will have an internal temperature of about 145°F). For the slaw, combine the watercress, cucumber, jicama, and alfalfa sprouts in a bowl. Now combine ½ teaspoon of both pepper and salt, 2 teaspoons of lime juice, and 2 tablespoons of extra virgin oil in a small bowl. Drizzle it over slaw and toss together to combine.

Nutritional value: Calories: 320 kcal Protein: 44g
Carbohydrate: 10g
Fat: 11 g

Cucumber-Basil Salsa on Halibut Pouches

Preparation Time: 10 minutes **Cooking Time:**
17 minutes **Servings:** 4
Ingredients:

- 1 lime, thinly sliced into 8 pieces
- 2 cups mustard greens, stems removed
- 2 teaspoon olive oil
- 4 – 5 radishes trimmed and quartered
- 4 4-oz skinless halibut filets - 4 large fresh basil leaves
- Cayenne pepper to taste – optional
- Pepper and salt to taste
- Salsa Ingredients: - 1 ½ cups diced cucumber
- 1 ½ finely chopped fresh basil leaves
- 2 teaspoon fresh lime juice - Pepper and salt to taste

Directions:
Preheat oven to 400oF.
Prepare parchment papers by making 4 pieces of 15 x 12-inch rectangles. Lengthwise, fold in half and unfold pieces on the table. Season halibut fillets with pepper, salt and cayenne—if using cayenne. Just to the right of the fold, place ½ cup of mustard greens. Add a basil leaf on center of mustard greens and topped with 1 lime slice. Around the greens, layer ¼ of the radishes. Drizzle with ½ teaspoon of oil, season with pepper and salt. Top it with a slice of halibut fillet. Just as you would make a calzone, fold parchment paper over your filling and crimp the edges of the parchment paper beginning from one end to the other end. To seal the end of the crimped parchment paper, pinch it. Repeat process to remaining ingredients until you have 4 pieces of parchment papers filled with halibut and greens. Place pouches in a pan and bake in the oven until halibut is flaky, around 15 to 17 minutes. While waiting for halibut pouches to cook, make your salsa by mixing all salsa ingredients in a medium bowl. Once halibut is cooked, remove from oven and make a tear on top. Be careful of the steam as it is very hot. Equally divide salsa and spoon ¼ of salsa on top of halibut through the slit you have created.
Nutritional value: Calories: 335.4 kcal Protein: 20.2g Fat: 16.3gCarbs: 22.1g

Chapter 6:

Lean and Green Chicken and Turkey Recipes

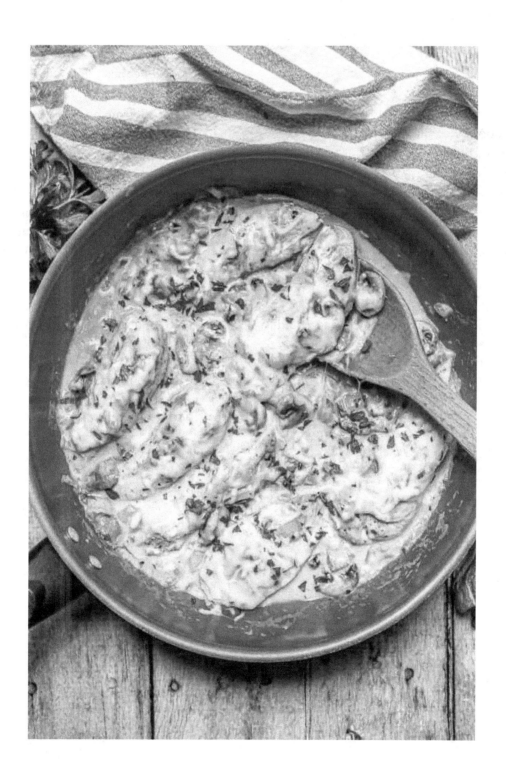

Instant Pot Chipotle Chicken & Cauliflower Rice Bowls

Preparation Time: 10 minutes
Cooking Time: 20 minutes
Servings: 4
Ingredients:

- ⅓ cup of salsa
- 1 quantity of 14.5 ounce of can fire-roasted diced tomatoes
- 1 canned chipotle pepper + 1 teaspoon sauce
- ½ teaspoon of dried oregano
- 1 teaspoon of cumin
- 1 ½ lb. of boneless, skinless chicken breast
- ¼ teaspoon of salt
- 1 cup of reduced-fat shredded Mexican cheese blend
- 4 cups of frozen riced cauliflower
- ½ medium-sized avocado, sliced

Directions:

1. Combine the first ingredients in a blender and blend until they become smooth
2. Place chicken inside your instant pot, and pour the sauce over it. Cover the lid and close the pressure valve. Set it to 20 minutes at high temperature. Let the pressure release on its own before opening. Remove the piece and the chicken and then add it back to the sauce.
3. Microwave the riced cauliflower according to the directions on the package
4. To serve: divide the riced cauliflower, cheese, avocado, and chicken equally among the 4 bowls.

Nutritional value:
Calories: 287 kcal
Protein: 35 g
Carbohydrate: 19 g
Fat: 12 g

Sheet Pan Chicken Fajita Lettuce Wraps

Preparation Time: 15 minutes
Cooking Time: 30 minutes
Servings: 2
Ingredients:

- 1 pounds chicken breast, thinly sliced into strips
- 2 teaspoon olive oil
- 2 bell peppers, thinly sliced into strips
- 2 teaspoon fajita seasoning
- 6 leaves from a romaine heart
- ½ lime, juiced
- ¼ cup plain of non-fat Greek yogurt

Directions:

- Preheat the oven to about 400°F
- Combine all of the ingredients except for the lettuce in a large plastic bag that can be resealed. Mix very well to coat the vegetables and the chicken with oil with the seasoning evenly.
- Spread the contents of the bag evenly on a foil-lined baking sheet. Bake it for about 25–30 minutes, until the chicken is thoroughly cooked.
- Serve on lettuce leaves and topped with Greek yogurt if you like

Nutritional value:
Calories: 387 k cal
Fat: 6 g
Carbohydrate: 14 g
Protein: 18 g

Lean and Green Stir Fry Chicken
Preparation Time: 5 minutes
Cooking Time: 25 minutes
Servings: 2
Ingredients:

- ½ cup chicken broth, low sodium
- 12 ounces skinless chicken breasts, cut into strips
- 1 cup red bell pepper, seeded and chopped
- 8 ounces (1 cup) broccoli, cut into florets
- One teaspoon crushed red pepper

Directions:

1. Place a small amount of chicken broth in a saucepan. Heat over medium flame and stir in the chicken. Water sauté the chicken for at least 5 minutes while stirring constantly.
2. Add the rest of the ingredients and stir.
3. Cover the pan with a lid and cook for another 5 minutes.

Nutritional value:
Calories per serving: 137 kcal
Protein: 15g
Carbs: 15.4g
Fat: 1.2g
Sugar: 0.6g

Lean and Green Garlic Chicken with Zoodles
Preparation Time: 5 minutes
Cooking Time: 10 minutes
Servings: 5
Ingredients:

- 1 ½ pound boneless and skinless chicken breasts, it should be cut into bite-sized pieces
- 6 slices sun-dried tomatoes
- 1 teaspoon chopped garlic
- 1 cup low fat plain Greek yogurt
- ½ cup chicken broth, low sodium
- ½ teaspoon garlic powder
- ½ teaspoon Italian seasoning
- 1 cup spinach, chopped
- 1 ½ cup zucchini, cut into thin noodles

Directions:

1. Place two tablespoons of water in a pan and heat over low-medium heat. Sauté the chicken for 3 minutes while constantly stirring until the sides are slightly golden.
2. Add in the tomatoes and garlic and stir for another 3 minutes. Add in the yogurt, chicken broth, garlic powder, and Italian seasoning. Cover the pan with its lid and just wait for it to simmer for at least 7 minutes.
3. Lastly, add in the spinach. Cook for another 2 minutes.
4. Place the zucchini noodles in a deep dish and pour over the chicken. Toss the noodles to soak with the sauce.
5. Serve immediately.

Nutritional value:
Calories per serving: 205kcal
Protein: 33.3g Carbs: 6g Fat: 2g Sugar: 1.2g

Lean and Green Crunchy Chicken Tacos

Preparation Time: 5 minutes
Cooking Time: 10 minutes **Servings:** 4
Ingredients:

- ½ cup low sodium chicken stock
- 2 chicken breasts, minced
- 1 red onion, chopped
- 1 garlic clove, minced
- 3 plum tomatoes, chopped
- 1 teaspoon cumin powder
- 1 teaspoon cinnamon powder
- 1 teaspoon ground coriander
- 1 red onion, chopped
- ½ red chili, chopped
- 1 tablespoon lemon juice
- 1 ripe avocado
- 1 cucumber, sliced into thick rounds

Directions:

1. Place a tablespoon of chicken stock in a pan and heat over medium heat. Sauté the chicken, onion, garlic, and tomatoes for 4 minutes or until the tomatoes have wilted.
2. Season with cumin, cinnamon, and coriander. Lessen the heat to low and cook for another 5 minutes. Set aside and allow it to cool.
3. In a bowl, mix together the onion, chili, lemon juice, and mashed avocado. It is the salsa.
4. Scoop the salsa and top on sliced cucumber. Top with cooked chicken.

Nutritional value:
Calories per serving: 313 kcal
Protein: 31.8g
Carbs: 14.9 g
Fat: 3.8g

Lean and Green Chicken Chili

Preparation Time: 5 minutes
Cooking Time: 45 minutes
Servings: 6
Ingredients:

- 1-pound boneless skinless chicken breast, chopped
- 1teaspoon ground cumin
- 1 cup chopped poblano pepper
- ½ cup chopped onion
- 1 garlic clove, minced
- 2 cups low-sodium chicken broth
- 1 cup rehydrated pinto beans
- 1 cup chopped tomatoes
- 2 tablespoons minced cilantro

Directions:

1. Make sure to put all the ingredients except the cilantro in a pressure cooker.
2. Close the lid and set it to the sealing position.
3. Cook on high for 45 minutes until the beans are soft.
4. Garnish with cilantro before serving.

Nutritional value:
Calories per serving: 229 kcal
Protein: 26.1g
Carbs: 23.9g
Fat: 2g
Sugar: 2.2g

Tomato Braised Cauliflower with Chicken

Preparation Time: 10 minutes
Cooking Time: 30 minutes
Servings: 4
Ingredients:

- 4 garlic cloves, sliced
- 3 scallions, to be trimmed and cut into 1 inch pieces
- ¼ teaspoon dried oregano
- ¼ teaspoon crushed red pepper flakes
- 4 ½ cups cauliflower
- 1 ½ cups diced canned tomatoes
- 1 cup fresh basil, gently torn
- ½ teaspoon each pepper and salt, divided
- 1 ½ teaspoon olive oil
- 1 ½ pounds boneless, skinless chicken breasts

Directions:

1. Get a saucepan and combine the garlic, scallions, oregano, crushed red pepper, cauliflower, and tomato, and add ¼ cup of water. Get everything boil together and add ¼ teaspoon of pepper and salt for seasoning, then cover the pot with a lid. Let it simmer for 10 minutes and stir as often as possible until you observe that the cauliflower is tender. Now, wrap up the seasoning with the remaining ¼ teaspoon of pepper and salt.
2. Toss the chicken breast with oil (olive prefebrably) and let it roast in the oven with the heat of 450°F for 20 minutes and an internal temperature of 165°F. Allow the chicken to rest for like 10 minutes.
3. Now slice the chicken, and serve on a bed of tomato braised cauliflower.

Nutritional value: Calories: 290 kcal Fat: 10 g Carbohydrate: 13 g Protein: 38 g

Lemon Garlic Oregano Chicken with Asparagus

Preparation Time: 5 minutes **Cooking Time:** 40 minutes **Servings:** 4
Ingredients:

- 1 small lemon, juiced (this should be about 2 tablespoons of lemon juice)
- 1 ¾ pounds bone-in, skinless chicken thighs
- 2 tablespoon fresh oregano, minced
- 2 cloves garlic, minced - 2 pounds asparagus, trimmed
- ¼ teaspoon each or less for black pepper and salt

Directions:

1. Preheat the oven to about 350°F.
2. Put the chicken in a medium-sized bowl. Now, add the garlic, oregano, lemon juice, pepper, and salt and toss them together to combine.
3. Roast the chicken in the airfryer until it reaches an internal temperature of 165°F in about 40 minutes. Once the chicken thighs have been cooked, remove and keep aside to rest.
4. Now, steam the asparagus on a stovetop or in a microwave to the desired doneness. Serve asparagus with the roasted chicken thighs.

Nutritional value: Calories: 350 kcal   Fat: 10 g Carbohydrate: 10 g   Protein: 32 g

Sophie Haye

Grilled Chicken Power Bowl With Green Goddess Dressing

Preparation Time: 15 minutes
Cooking Time: 45 minutes
Servings: 4
Ingredients:

- 1 ½ boneless, skinless chicken breasts
- 1/4 teaspoon each salt & pepper
- 1 cup rice or cubed kabocha squash
- 1 cup diced zucchini
- 1 cup rice yellow summer squash
- 1 cup rice broccoli
- 8 cherry tomatoes, halved
- 4 radishes, sliced thin
- 1 cup shredded red cabbage
- 1/4 cup hemp or pumpkin seeds

For the Green Goddess Dressing:

- 1/2 cup low-fat plain Greek yogurt
- 1 cup fresh basil
- 1 clove garlic
- 4 tablespoon lemon juice
- 1/4 tsp. each salt & pepper

Directions:

1. Preheat oven to 350°F. Season chicken with salt and pepper.
2. Roast chicken about 10–12 minutes until it reaches a temperature of 165°F.
3. When done, dismiss from oven and set aside to rest, about 5 minutes.
4. Cut into bite-sized pieces and keep warm.
5. While the chicken rests, steam the riced kabocha squash, yellow summer squash, zucchini, and broccoli in a covered microwave-proof bowl about 5 minutes till tender.
6. For the dressing, arrange the ingredients in a blender and puree till smooth.
7. To serve, put an equal amount of the riced veggie mixture into four individual serving bowls.
8. Add an equal amount of cherry tomatoes, radishes, and shredded cabbage to each bowl along with a quarter of the chicken and one tablespoon of seeds.
9. Drizzle dressing on top.

Nutritional value:
Calories: 300 kcal
Protein: 43 g
Carbohydrates: 12 g
Fat: 10 g

Chicken Strips

Preparation Time: 10 minutes
Cooking Time: 50 minutes
Servings: 3
Ingredients:

- 1 Medifast Snack Cracker Pack
- 6 Ounces breast, cut into strips
- 2 Pockets. Walden Farms Dressing Salad, every taste

Directions:

1. Preheat oven to 350 ° C. Pulse 1 packet of Medifast Snack Crackers in a food processor.
2. These must be pulsed into excellent crumbs.
3. Dip chicken SEED gently into dressing for Walden Farms Salad.
4. Shake off the dressing.
5. In essence, you just want to get the chicken wet so that the crumbs can stick to them.
6. Press the strips of chicken over the crumbs.
7. Take your time and get sweet, coated chicken.
8. Then spray Pam or some other non-stick cooking spray to a baking sheet.
9. Place the chicken on the sheet and bake within 30-40 minutes.

Nutritional value:
Fat: 25.7 g
Fiber: 2.2 g
Protein: 35.4 g

Chicken Stir Fry

Preparation Time: 10 minutes
Cooking Time: 10 minutes
Servings: 2
Ingredients:

- Boneless and skinless breast chicken
- 1 cup each chopped red bell pepper and green bell pepper
- 1 cup broccoli slaw
- 1 teaspoon of crushed red pepper
- ½ cup chicken broth
- 2 tablespoon soy sauce

Directions:

1. Add chopped red and green bell pepper into the chicken broth, add the broccoli slaw also.
2. Next, add your soy sauce, red pepper, and the boneless chicken (shredded).
3. Stir and allow to cook for a few minutes, do this until the peppers are tender and your delicacy is ready.

Nutritional value:
Calories 137.0 kcal
Fats 1.2 g
Cholesterol: 27.5 mg
Sodium: 873.4 mg
Total Carbs: 15.4 g
Dietary Fiber: 7.0 g   Protein: 15.1 g

Chicken Paella

Preparation Time: 5 minutes
Cooking Time: 25 minutes
Servings: 8
Ingredients:

- ¼ teaspoon each (or as desired) of pepper and salt
- 1 cup green beans, which are to be cut into ¼ inch pieces
- 1 cup diced tomatoes
- Pinch saffron (optional)
- 4 cups cauliflower rice
- 1 scallion should be trimmed and minced
- 2 garlic cloves should be minced
- 1 ½ pound of boneless skinless chicken breasts that is to be diced into bite-sized pieces.
- 2 ounces of seitan chorizo crumbles, like Upton's Natural Vegan Chorizo Seitan Crumbles
- 4 teaspoon of canola oil

Directions:

1. Get a skillet, pour the oil and heat with medium-high heat, then cook the chicken and add the chorizo crumbles until they become brown but not thoroughly cooked.
2. Add the scallions and garlic and let it sweat for about 2 minutes.
3. Finally, add the saffron (if you decide to use it), green beans, tomatoes, and cauliflower rice to the paella. You will need to cook for about 10 minutes and season with pepper and salt.
4. Serve while hot.

Nutritional value:
Calories: 300 kcal
Protein: 41g
Carbohydrate: 13g
Fat: 10g

Pesto Zucchini Noodles with Grilled Chicken

Preparation Time: 5 minutes
Cooking Time: 25 minutes
Servings: 8
Ingredients:

- ½ teaspoon crushed red pepper flakes (optional)
- 2 cups cherry tomatoes, which needs to be halved
- 1 ½ pounds grilled boneless skinless chicken breast, cubed or cut into little strips
- 1 ½ pounds zucchini, sliced, cut, or "spiralized" into noodle-like strands (it should give about 4 cups of Zucchini noodles)
- Cooking spray
- 1/3 ounces pine nuts
- ½ cup parmesan cheese, to be divided
- ½ cup chopped fresh basil
- 1/3 cup reduced-fat Italian salad dressing

Directions:

1. To make the pesto, combine the basil, pine nuts, 2 tablespoons. of parmesan cheese, and salad dressing in a food processor. Blend very well until they become smooth.
2. Get a lightly greased skillet, put the zucchini noodles, and place it over medium heat. Cook until the zucchini noodles become tender in about 3-5 minutes. Next is to stir in the remaining parmesan cheese and pesto and remove it from the heat.
3. Add tomatoes, and you can top it with grilled chicken and garnish with your crushed red pepper flakes.

Nutritional value:
Calories: 380 kcal
Protein: 58g Carbohydrate: 12 g
Fat: 12g

Chicken Parmesan with Zucchini Noodles & Marinara

Preparation Time: 5 minutes
Cooking Time: 25 minutes
Servings: 4
Ingredients:

- ½ cup almond flour
- ½ teaspoon each pepper and salt. Divided
- 1 ¾ pound boneless, skinless chicken breasts
- 2 teaspoons large flake nutritional yeast
- ½ teaspoon dried oregano
- 15 ounces can petite diced tomatoes
- 2 scallions, chopped
- 2 garlic cloves, minced
- 2 medium zucchinis, sliced, cut, or "spiralized" into noodle-like strands

Directions:

1. Preheat the oven to 400°F.
2. Combine the nutritional yeast and almond flour in a medium-sized bowl. Season the chicken breast using pepper & salt, and then coat it sides with almond mixture.
3. Bake for around 12-15 minutes or till the internal temperature becomes 165°F. Once it's cooked, remove the chicken from the oven and keep aside to rest.
4. While the chicken bakes, combine the tomatoes, scallions, garlic, and oregano in a pot and simmer on low for about 15-20 minutes.
5. Steam the zucchini noodles inside a steamer basket over boiling water on the stovetop for it to tender.
6. Serve zucchini noodles with marinara and chicken.

Nutritional value:
Calories: 360 kcal
Protein: 49 g
Carbohydrate: 16 g
Fat: 12g

Chicken Cacciatore

Preparation Time: 5 minutes
Cooking Time: 6 to 8 Hours
Servings: 4
Ingredients:

- ¼ teaspoon each pepper and salt
- ¼ cup fresh basil, to be chopped
- 1 large zucchini, cut, sliced, or "spiralized" into noddle-like strands
- 1 bay leaf
- Diced tomatoes
- 1 cup button mushrooms, to be halved
- 1 small bell pepper, the seeds, and membranes should be removed and chopped
- 2 scallions, to be minced
- 2 garlic cloves, to be minced
- 4 x 7 ounces raw bone-in skinless chicken thighs

Directions:

1. Combine the garlic, mushrooms, bell peppers, bay leaf, chicken, tomatoes, pepper, and salt in a slow cooker and set to low for 6-8 hours.
2. Just before you serve, stir in the basil and zucchini noodles; make sure to mix very well to combine.

Nutritional value:

Calories: 310 kcal
Protein: 38 g
Carbohydrate: 15 g
Fat: 12g

Cheesy Chicken Cauliflower Skillet

Preparation Time: 5 minutes
Cooking Time: 15 minutes
Servings: 4
Ingredients:

- 2 scallions, to be chopped
- ½ teaspoon dried oregano
- 8 ounces reduced-fat shredded mozzarella cheese
- 1, 12-ounces of can sliced chicken breast, to be drained
- ½ cup chicken broth
- 1 ½ cups sliced mushrooms
- 2 teaspoon olive oil
- 2 garlic cloves, to be minced
- 12 ounces bag frozen riced cauliflower

Directions:

1. You will need to cook the mushrooms, garlic, and cauliflower in oil for about 3-4 minutes. Pour the broth and wait for it to boil
2. Add the chicken, reduce the heat, and let it simmer for 4-5 minutes or until the vegetables are now tender and the chicken becomes cooked thoroughly. Then stir in oregano and mozzarella and top with scallions.

Nutritional value:

Calories: 380 kcal Protein: 58g
Carbohydrate: 12 g Fat: 12g

Sophie Haye

Chicken Casserole
Preparation Time: 15 minutes
Cooking Time: 40 minutes
Servings: 4
Ingredients:
- 1 pounds cooked chicken, shredded
- ¼ cup Greek yogurt
- 1 cup cheddar cheese, shredded
- ½ cup salsa
- 4 ounces cream cheese, softened
- 4 cups cauliflower florets
- ⅛ teaspoons black pepper
- ½ teaspoons kosher salt

Directions:
1. Add the cauliflower florets into the microwave-safe dish and cook for 10 minutes or until tender.
2. Add the cream cheese and microwave for 30 seconds more. Stir well.
3. Add the chicken, yogurt, cheddar cheese, salsa, pepper, and salt and stir everything well.
4. Preheat the oven to 375 F.
5. Bake in preheated oven for 20 minutes.
6. Serve hot and enjoy.

Nutritional value:
Calories 429 kcal
Fat 23 g   Carbs 6 g   Sugar 7 g
Protein 44 g
Cholesterol 149 mg

Chicken Broccoli Salad with Avocado Dressing
Preparation Time: 5 minutes
Cooking Time: 40 minutes
Servings: 6
Ingredients:
- 2 chicken breasts
- 1 pound broccoli, cut into florets
- 1 avocado, peeled and pitted
- ½ lemon, juiced
- 2 garlic cloves
- ¼ teaspoon chili powder
- ¼ teaspoon cumin powder
- Salt and pepper to taste

Directions:
1. Cook the chicken in a large pot of salty water.
2. Drain and cut the chicken into small cubes. Place in a salad bowl.
3. Add the broccoli and mix well.
4. Combine the avocado, lemon juice, garlic, chili powder, cumin powder, salt and pepper in a blender. Pulse until smooth.
5. Spoon the dressing over the salad and mix well.
6. Serve the salad fresh.

Nutritional value:
Calories: 195 kcal   Fat: 11 g
Protein: 14 g   Carbohydrates: 3 g

Herbed Roasted Chicken Breasts

Preparation Time: 5 minutes
Cooking Time: 50 minutes
Servings: 4
Ingredients:

- 2 tablespoons extra virgin olive oil
- 2 tablespoons chopped parsley
- 2 tablespoons chopped cilantro
- 1 teaspoon dried oregano
- 1 teaspoon dried basil
- 2 tablespoons lemon juice
- Salt and pepper to taste
- 4 chicken breasts

Directions:

1. Combine the oil, parsley, cilantro, oregano, basil, lemon juice, salt and pepper in a bowl.
2. Spread this mixture over the chicken and rub it well into the meat.
3. Place in a deep dish baking pan and cover with aluminum foil.
4. Cook in the preheated oven at 350°F for 20 minutes then remove the foil and cook for 25 additional minutes.
5. Serve the chicken warm and fresh with your favorite side dish.

Nutritional value:

Calories: 330 kcal   Fat: 15 g
Protein: 40.7 g   Carbohydrates: 1 g

Marinated Chicken Breasts

Preparation Time: 5 minutes **Cooking Time:** 2 hours **Servings:** 4
Ingredients:

- 4 chicken breasts
- Salt and pepper to taste
- 1 lemon, juiced
- 1 rosemary sprig
- 1 thyme sprig
- 2 garlic cloves, crushed
- 2 sage leaves
- 3 tablespoons extra virgin olive oil
- ½ cup buttermilk

Directions:

1. Boil the chicken with salt and pepper and place it in a resealable bag.
2. Add remaining ingredients and seal the bag.
3. Refrigerate for at least 1 hour.
4. After 1 hour, heat a roasting pan over medium heat, then place the chicken on the grill.
5. Cook on each side for 8-10 minutes or until juices are gone.
6. Serve the chicken warm with your favorite side dish.

Nutritional value:

Calories: 371 kcal   Fat: 21 g
Protein: 46 g   Carbohydrates: 2 g

Garlic Chicken Balls

Preparation Time: 15 minutes
Cooking Time: 10 minutes
Servings: 4
Ingredients:

- 2 cups ground chicken
- 1 teaspoon minced garlic
- 1 teaspoon dried dill
- 1/3 carrot, grated
- 1 egg, beaten
- 1 tablespoon olive oil
- ¼ cup coconut flakes
- ½ teaspoon salt

Directions:

- In a mixing bowl mix up together ground chicken, minced garlic, dried dill, carrot, egg, and salt.
- Stir the chicken mixture with the help of the fingertips until homogenous.
- Then make medium balls from the mixture.
- Coat every chicken ball in coconut flakes.
- Heat up olive oil in the skillet.
- Add chicken balls and cook them for 3 minutes each side. The cooked chicken balls will have a golden-brown color.

Nutritional value:
Calories 200 kcal Fat 11.5 g Fiber 0.6 g
Carbs 1.7 g Protein 21.9 g

Mediterranean Chicken Salad

Preparation Time: 5 minutes
Cooking Time: 25 minutes
Servings: 4
Ingredients:
For the Chicken:

- 1 ¾ pounds boneless, skinless chicken breast
- ¼ teaspoon each pepper and salt (or as desired)
- 1 ½ tablespoon butter, melted

For the Mediterranean salad:

- 1 cup of sliced cucumber
- 6 cups of romaine lettuce, that is torn or roughly chopped
- 10 pitted Kalamata olives
- 1 pint of cherry tomatoes
- ⅓ cup of reduced-fat feta cheese
- ¼ teaspoon each pepper and salt (or lesser)
- 1 small lemon, juiced (it should be about 2 tablespoons)

Directions:

1. Preheat the oven or grill to about 350°F.
2. Season the chicken with the salt, butter, and black pepper.
3. Roast or grill chicken until it reaches an internal temperature of 165°F (about 25 minutes.) Once your chicken breasts are cooked, remove and keep aside to rest for about 5 minutes before you slice it.
4. Combine all the salad ingredients you have and toss everything together very well
5. Serve the chicken with Mediterranean salad

Nutritional values:
Calories: 340 kcal Protein: 45g Carbohydrate: 9g

Riced Cauliflower & Curry Chicken

Preparation Time: 15 minutes
Cooking Time: 30 minutes
Servings: 6
Ingredients:

- 2 pounds chicken (4 breasts)
- 1 pack curry paste
- 3 tablespoons ghee (can substitute with butter)
- ½ cup heavy cream
- 1 head cauliflower (around 1 kg)

Directions:

1. In a large frying pan, melt the ghee.
2. Add the curry paste and mix together.
3. Once combined, add a cup of water and simmer for 5 minutes.
4. Add the chicken, cover the frying pan and simmer for 18 minutes.
5. Cut a cauliflower head into florets and blend it in a food processor to make the cauliflower rice.
6. When the chicken is cooked, add the cream and cook for an additional 7 minutes.
7. Serve!

Nutritional value:
Calories: 267 kcal
Carbs: 42 g Fat: 31 g
Protein: 34 g Fiber: 32 g

Blue Cheese Chicken Wedges

Preparation Time: 20 minutes
Cooking Time: 45 minutes
Servings: 4
Ingredients:

- Blue cheese dressing
- 2 tablespoons crumbled blue cheese
- 4 strips of bacon
- 2 chicken breasts (boneless)
- 3/4 cup of your favorite buffalo sauce

Directions:

1. Boil a large pot of salted water.
2. Add in the two chicken breasts to the pot and cook for 28 minutes.
3. Turn off the heat and let the chicken rest for 10 minutes. Using a fork, pull the chicken apart into strips.
4. Cook and cool the bacon strips and put them aside.
5. On a medium heat, combine the chicken and buffalo sauce. Stir until hot.
6. Add the blue cheese to the chicken and buffalo sauce. Top with the cooked bacon.
7. Serve and enjoy.

Nutritional value:
Calories: 309 kcal
Carbs: 27 g
Fat: 18 g
Protein: 34 g
Fiber: 29 g

Crispy Buffalo Chicken Bites
Preparation Time: 15 minutes
Cooking Time: 30 minutes
Servings: 1
Ingredients:
- 8 ounces cubed chicken breast
- 1 bag Medifast's Parmesan Cheese Puffs
- 2 tablespoons Frank's Red-Hot Sauce
- 2 tablespoons reduced-fat grated parmesan cheese
  Optional Sauce for Dipping:
- ½ tablespoons Frank's Hot Sauce
- 2 tablespoons Hidden Valley's Light Ranch Dressing

Directions:
1. Heat the oven at 350° F. Cover a baking tray using a layer of parchment baking paper.
2. Crush the parmesan puffs into a fine - bread-crumb consistency by hand or using a food processor. Combine the processed puffs with the parmesan cheese and pour it into a plastic zipper-type bag. Put it aside for now.
3. Slice the chicken breasts into approximately one-inch chunks. Combine the chicken with the hot sauce, mix it until it's well combined.
4. Toss the coated chicken into the zipper bag with the crumb mixture and shake until the chicken is completely covered.
5. Arrange the prepared cubes of chicken onto the baking tray and bake them for approximately 25 to 30 minutes.
6. Meanwhile, whisk the ranch dressing and hot sauce until it's well combined. Serve with chicken bites.

Nutritional value: Calories: 4030 kcal Protein: 454.68 gFat: 59 .09 g Carbohydrates: 403.85 g

Glazed Ginger Chicken and Green
Preparation Time: 5 minutes
Cooking Time: 20-35 minutes
Servings: 4
Ingredients
- 1 tablespoon Toasted Sesame Ginger Seasoning
- 1 ½ pounds boneless skinless chicken (breasts or thighs)
- Nonstick cooking spray
- ¼ cup low sodium soy sauce
- ½ cup water
- 4 cups fresh green beans, ends snipped

Directions:
1. Preheat the oven to 350°F.
2. In a medium bowl, add the chicken, ginger seasoning, and soy sauce. Mix to combine. Marinate at room temperature.
3. Spray a large baking sheet with cooking spray; add the chicken mixture and spread evenly.
4. Place the sheet on the middle rack in the oven and roast for 20 minutes. If desired, soak the chicken with the liquid from the bowl (2-4 tablespoons) one to three times while roasting.
5. Remove the baking sheet from the oven.
6. Add the green beans (in the bowl) and water; cover the pan with aluminum foil and bake for 10 to 15 more minutes.
7. Remove the pan and stir the beans. Bake for an additional 5 to 7 minutes, or until the beans are tender.
8. Serve and sprinkle with some fresh ground pepper.

Nutritional value:
Calories: 259 kcal   Protein: 41.77 g
Fat: 6.23 g
Carbohydrates: 8.04 g
Calcium: 77 mg
Magnesium: 86 mg
Phosphorus: 435 mg

Slow-Cooked Chicken with Fire Roasted Tomatoes

Preparation Time: 10 minutes
Cooking Time: 3 hours and 10 minutes
Servings: 4
Ingredients

- 1 ½ pounds boneless, skinless chicken breast
- 15 ounces can fire roasted tomatoes (no added sugar)
- 2 tablespoons salt
- 2 tablespoons ground black pepper
- 2 tablespoons oil
- 2 tablespoons sage
- 2 tablespoons black pepper
- 2 tablespoons onion and garlic

Directions:

1. Add the oil and chicken breasts to the slow cooker.
2. Pour all of the spices over the chicken and put the lid on.
3. Cook on high heat for 3 hours.
4. Add fire roasted tomatoes and cook for 10 additional minutes.
5. Using a handheld blender, or an upright blender, blend 6 tablespoon of the liquid into the chicken.
6. Remove the chicken and put on the plate.
7. Shred chicken into smaller pieces using two forks.
8. Serve over white or brown rice.

Nutritional value:
Calories: 400 kcal
Protein: 17.7 g
Fat: 17.12 g
Carbohydrates: 45.65 g
Calcium: 131 mg
Magnesium: 62 mg
Phosphorus: 188 mg

Sweet & Smoky Pulled Chicken

Preparation Time: 10 minutes
Cooking Time: 20 minutes **Servings:** 6
Ingredients

- 1.65 pounds chicken breasts, skinless and boneless
- 13.5 ounces unsweetened tomato sauce
- 3.5 ounces apple cider vinegar
- 3 tablespoon Swerve or Erythritol
- 1 tablespoon molasses (optional)
- 1 teaspoon sea salt
- 1 teaspoon black pepper
- 1 teaspoon garlic powder
- ¼ teaspoon cayenne pepper, or to taste
- 1 tablespoon smoked paprika
- 3 tablespoon coconut aminos
- ¼ cup extra virgin olive oil
- 1 cup sour cream, full-fat yogurt or creme fraiche to serve (optional)

Directions:

1. In a large bowl, place the chicken breasts and cover them with the tomato sauce. Add the ground or whole peppercorns, salt, black pepper, and garlic powder. Whisk to combine and transfer to the slow cooker. Whisk again to cover everything and let it cook on low heat for 5 hours.
2. Cook the rice according to the package direction and transfer to a large bowl. Add the sour cream, coconut cream, and Swerve. Whisk until combined.
3. Finely mince the fresh parsley. Mix the parsley and the smoked paprika with the rice.
4. To serve, put the rice on the chicken and top with the sour cream, yogurt or creme fraiche.

Nutritional value:

Calories: 2924 kcal	Protein: 85.2 g
Fat: 27.19 g	Magnesium: 347
Carbohydrates: 515.51 g	Phosphorus: 1475 mg
Calcium: 578 mg mg	

Finger Licking BBQ Crock Pot Chicken

Preparation Time: 10 minutes
Cooking Time: 6 hours **Servings:** 4
Ingredients

- 1 ⅓ pounds Boneless Skinless Chicken (thigh or breasts)
- 1 tablespoon Stacey Hawkins Honey BBQ Seasoning
- 1 tablespoon Stacey Hawkins Garlic & Spring Onion Seasoning
- 1 tablespoon Phoenix Sunrise Seasoning

Directions:

1. In a slow cooker, mix all of the seasonings together.
2. Remove any fat and skin from the chicken and cut it into equally-sized pieces.
3. Add the chicken pieces to the seasonings in the slow cooker.
4. Drizzle 2 tablespoons of honey BBQ over the chicken pieces. Mix together.
5. Cook for 6 hours on low setting.
6. Before serving, add ¼ cup BBQ sauce to the chicken in the slow cooker.
7. Mix thoroughly and cook for 5 minutes on high heat to let the BBQ sauce cook into the chicken.

Nutritional value:
Calories: 400 kcal
Protein: 17.7 g
Carbohydrates: 45.65 g
Magnesium: 62 mg
mg

Fat: 17.12 g
Calcium: 131 mg
Phosphorus: 188

Chicken with Garlic and Spring Onion Cream

Preparation Time: 5 minutes
Cooking Time: 15 minutes**Servings:** 4
Ingredients:

- 6 medium chicken breasts
- 3 tablespoons butter or 3 tablespoons margarine
- 2 tablespoons all-purpose flour
- ⅓ cup chopped green onion
- ¾ cup chicken broth
- ¼ teaspoon salt
- Pepper
- 1 or 2 tablespoon Dijon mustard to taste
- 1 cup plain yogurt

Directions:

1. Heat a large skillet, add 1 tablespoon butter. Add the chicken breasts to the pan. Cook for 10 minutes on medium heat, until browned on both sides. Remove and set aside on a plate.
2. On a chopping board cut the chicken breasts into thin strips.
3. Melt 2 tablespoons butter in the same skillet. Add in flour and cook for 2 minutes, stirring constantly. Gradually add the chicken broth, mustard, salt and pepper. (For a thicker sauce, add 2 tablespoons of cornstarch dissolved in ½ cup cold water.)
4. Blend in the yogurt. Add the chicken strips and green onion. Cook until sauce bubbles and thickens, stirring occasionally.
5. Serve with plain white rice or boiled potatoes.

Nutritional value:
Calories: 1172 kcal   Phosphorus: 1073 mg
Protein: 132.83 g
Fat: 63.49 g
Carbohydrates: 9.7 g
Calcium:162 mg
Magnesium: 155 mg

Cheesy Chicken Caprese

Preparation Time: 15 minutes **Cooking Time:** 15 minutes **Servings:** 2

Ingredients:

- 2 boneless, skinless chicken breasts, pounded to uniform thickness
- ½ cup good-quality balsamic vinegar
- 1 cup grape or cherry tomatoes, halved
- ⅓ cup sliced fresh mozzarella
- fresh basil - salt - pepper
- optional: liquid stevia

Directions:

1. Preheat oven to 350°F with the rack in the center.
2. Pour balsamic vinegar into a 9×13 inch baking dish. Halve the chicken breasts horizontally, and place the chicken pieces into the baking dish.
3. Brush the chicken with a small amount of balsamic vinegar. Combine the salt, pepper and the optional liquid stevia to create a paste, and season each piece of chicken with the paste.
4. Bake the chicken for 15 minutes, until the chicken is opaque and the balsamic vinegar is reduced and thickened. On the stove top over medium high heat, sauté the sliced cherry tomatoes in a small amount of balsamic vinegar for a few minutes, until they begin to soften.
5. Place a halved chicken breast on top of the sliced tomatoes, followed by the fresh mozzarella cheese and a pinch of fresh basil. Serve immediately.

Nutritional value: Calories: 511 kcal Protein: 82.6 g Fat: 11.66 g Phosphorus, P1233 mg Carbohydrates: 16.93 g Calcium, Ca133 mg Magnesium, Mg131 mg

Creamy Skillet Chicken and Asparagus

Preparation Time: 5 minutes **Cooking Time:** 20 minutes **Servings:** 4

Ingredients:

- 1 ½ tablespoon extra-virgin olive oil
- 4 (16 ounces) boneless skinless chicken breasts
- salt and fresh ground pepper to taste
- 2 teaspoons Italian Seasoning
- 1 tablespoon butter
- 1 pound asparagus stalks trimmed and cut into thirds
- 1 yellow onion sliced
- 1 cup fat free half & half (you can also use low fat evaporated milk)
- ½ tablespoon all-purpose flour
- ⅓ cup grated Parmesan
- 1 lemon, juiced - 3 Garlic cloves minced
- salt and fresh ground pepper to taste
- lemon slices - chopped parsley - freshly grated parmesan

Directions:

1. Heat big nonstick omelet pan over medium high heat. Add the olive oil and swirl. Season the chicken with salt and pepper and the Italian seasoning. Add the chicken to the pan and sauté until tops are brown (about 4 minutes,) then flip and cook for another 4–5 minutes, or until golden. Remove the chicken from pan and keep warm. Add the butter, the asparagus, and the onion to the pan, and sauté until the asparagus are tender (about 4 mins.) Season the asparagus. Sprinkle in the flour, stirring constantly, until the mixture is homogenized and bubbly. Gradually add the 1/2 cup of half and half, stirring constantly, then add parmesan cheese, garlic, lemon juice, salt and pepper. Cook until sauce thickens (about 2 minutes.) Taste and adjust seasoning. Stir in the rest of the half and half. Add chicken back into the pan to reheat and toss together with the sauce. Remove from heat. Serve and garnish with the lemon slices, parsley and the parmesan. You can also garnish it with your favorite spaghetti sauce.

Nutritional value: Calories: 703 kcal Protein: 110.07 g Fat: 18.54 g
Carbohydrates: 19.52 g Calcium, Ca190 mg Magnesium, Mg171 mg

Kale Slaw and Strawberry Salad + Poppyseed Dressing

Preparation Time: 10 minutes
Cooking Time: 20 minutes
Servings: 2
Ingredients:
- 8 ounces chicken breast, sliced and baked
- 1 cup kale, chopped
- 1 cup slaw mix (cabbage, broccoli slaw, carrots mixed)
- ¼ cup slivered almonds
- 1 cup strawberries, sliced
  For the dressing:
- 1 tablespoon light mayonnaise
- Dijon mustard
- 1 tablespoon olive oil
- 1 tablespoon apple cider vinegar
- ½ teaspoon lemon juice
- 1 tablespoon honey
- ¼ teaspoon onion powder
- ¼ teaspoon garlic powder
- Poppyseeds

Directions:
1. Whisk the dressing ingredients together until well mixed, then leave it to cool in the fridge.
2. Slice the chicken breasts.
3. Divide 2 bowls of spinach, slaw, and strawberries.
4. Cover with a sliced breast of chicken (4 ounces each), then scatter with almonds.
5. Divide the salad over the chicken and drizzle the dressing.

Nutritional value:
Calories: 340 kcal
Fats: 13.6 g
Saturated Fat: 6.2 g

Chicken Zucchini Noodles
Preparation Time: 20 minutes
Cooking Time: 5 minutes
Servings: 2
Ingredients:
- 1 large zucchini, spiralized
- 1 chicken breast, skinless & boneless
- ½ tablespoon jalapeno, minced
- 2 garlic cloves, minced
- ½ teaspoon ginger, minced
- ½ tablespoon fish sauce
- 2 tablespoon coconut cream
- ½ tablespoon honey
- ½ lime juice
- 1 tablespoon peanut butter
- 1 carrot, chopped
- 2 tablespoon cashews, chopped
- ¼ cup fresh cilantro, chopped
- 1 tablespoon olive oil
- Pepper
- Salt

Directions:
1. Heat the olive oil in a pan over medium-high heat.
2. Season the chicken breast with pepper and salt. Once the oil is hot then add the chicken breast into the pan and cook for 3-4 minutes per side or until cooked.
3. Remove chicken breast from pan. Shred chicken breast with a fork and set aside.
4. In a small bowl, mix together the peanut butter, jalapeno, garlic, ginger, fish sauce, coconut cream, honey, and lime juice. Set aside.
5. In a large mixing bowl, combine together the spiralized zucchini, carrots, cashews, cilantro, and shredded chicken.
6. Pour peanut butter mixture over zucchini noodles and mix to combine.
7. Serve immediately and enjoy.

Nutritional value:
Calories: 353 kcal   Fat: 21 g
Carbs: 20.5 g   Sugar: 8 g
Protein: 25 g   Cholesterol: 54 mg

Zucchini Pappardelle with Sausage

Preparation Time: 5 minutes **Cooking Time:** 15 minutes **Servings:** 4

Ingredients

- 1 ½ pounds lean turkey or chicken sausage, Italian seasoned (your choice of sweet or hot)
- 2 cups chopped tomatoes
- 1 Tablespoon Stacey Hawkins' Garlic and Spring Onion Seasoning
- 4 Cups noodles made from fresh zucchini (about 3 zucchinis, 8 long)
- 4 teaspoons Olive Oil
- 1 teaspoon Stacey Hawkins' Dash of Desperation Seasoning

Directions:

1. Wash and gently dry the zucchini. Cut it lengthwise into spaghetti sized strips; using vegetable peeler, peel the zucchini into thin shreds. Transfer it to a salad spinner. Sprinkle with 1 teaspoon of olive oil and Dash of Desperation Seasoning until it's covered. In a skillet, brown sausage; drain fat and transfer it to a large pot. Add 2 teaspoons of olive oil, chopped tomatoes and Stacey Hawkins Garlic and Spring Onion Seasoning. Cook over high heat until tomatoes are softened, for about 5 minutes.

2. Fill a large pot generously with salted water. Bring water to boil and cook the zucchini pasta for 7 minutes. While you are cooking it, add the sausage, tomato and seasoning combination to the zucchini pasta and cook together on medium heat.

3. Use tongs to submerge zucchini noodles one at a time into a large pot of boiling water with 1 teaspoon of olive oil stirred in. Once done, strain it along with other ingredients.

4. Preheat the oven to 350°F. Transfer all ingredients to a large casserole or baking dish and mix thoroughly. Top dish with fresh grated Parmesan cheese. Bake in a preheated oven until the cheese is golden brown and it is bubbly, for about 15 minutes.

5. This dish is equally delicious served either hot or cold. Serve in a bowl with a little of the pasta water stir into it.

Nutritional value: Calories: 801 kcal Protein: 33.31 g Fat: 51.13 g Carbohydrates: 49.95 g Calcium: 58 mg Magnesium: 41 mg Phosphorus: 321 mg

Asian Stir Fry

Preparation Time: 15 minutes
Cooking Time: 10 minutes **Servings:** 4

Ingredients:

- 1 teaspoon olive oil
- 1 teaspoon low sodium soy sauce
- 1 lemon wedge
- 7 ounces of boneless, skinless chicken breast (Split into strips)
- ¾ cups broccoli blossoms
- ½ cups chestnuts, sliced
- ¼ cup red bell pepper
- ¼ cup fresh water
- Ground potatoes to taste

Directions:

1. Prepare the chicken and veggies.
2. Add oil, soy sauce and lime wedge juice, in a medium to large saucepan.
3. Put on medium heat, then add the chicken. Cook chicken over regularly, tossing or stirring.
4. Remove the chicken from the saucepan and put it aside.
5. Add water to the saucepan and stir until the water gets warm.
6. Next add the vegetables, and mix well.
7. Put the lid on and let it cook for 5-7 minutes, until the vegetables are almost tender.
8. Remove the lid and add the chicken, cook over medium-high to high heat until the vegetables are cooked and the liquid is evaporated completely

Nutritional value:

Carbohydrates: 13 g Protein: 4 g Fat: 8 g
Sodium: 485 mg Potassium: 392 mg
Fiber: 2 g

Turkey Taco
Preparation Time: 10 minutes
Cooking Time: 20 minutes **Servings:** 4
Ingredients:

- 2 pre-made rolls ($\frac{1}{3}$ lean, 1 $\frac{1}{3}$ condiment)
- 4 ounces of turkey ($\frac{2}{3}$ thin) white meat leftover from Thanksgiving!
- 2 Tablespoons of salad with cranberry ($\frac{1}{4}$ snack, 1/8th green)
- Shredded laitoux

Directions:

1. Toast the buns with 2.
2. Next put 1 tablespoon of sugar-free cranberry salad, then 2 ounces of turkey and top with a little shredded lettuce.
3. Fold up like a taco, and eat. 2 Tacos is equivalent to 1 serving.
4. 1 Lean, 1/3 seasoning, 1/4 snack, 1/8 orange.
5. You will need to combine this with a green to make it a lean and nutritious meal in its entirety.

Nutritional value:
Protein: 17.6 g
Carbohydrates: 4.8 g
Fats: 7.2 g
Cholesterol: 62.7 mg

Taco Zucchini Boats
Preparation Time: 20 minutes
Cooking Time: 55 minutes **Servings:** 4
Ingredients:

- 4 medium zucchinis, cut in half lengthwise
- $\frac{1}{4}$ cup fresh cilantro, chopped
- $\frac{1}{2}$ cup cheddar cheese, shredded
- $\frac{1}{4}$ cup water
- 4 ounces tomato sauce
- 2 tablespoon bell pepper, mined
- $\frac{1}{2}$ small onion, minced
- $\frac{1}{2}$ teaspoon oregano
- 1 teaspoon paprika
- 1 teaspoon chili powder
- 1 teaspoon cumin
- 1 teaspoon garlic powder
- 1 lb. lean ground turkey
- $\frac{1}{2}$ cup salsa - 1 teaspoon kosher salt

Directions:

- Preheat the oven to 400 °F.
- Add $\frac{1}{4}$ cup of salsa in the bottom of the baking dish.
- Using a spoon hollow out the center of the zucchini halves.
- Chop the scooped-out flesh of zucchini and set aside $\frac{3}{4}$ of a cup chopped flesh.
- Add the zucchini halves in the boiling water and cook for 1 minute. Remove zucchini halves from water.
- Add the ground turkey in a large pan and cook until meat is no longer pink. Add spices and mix well.
- Add reserved zucchini flesh, water, tomato sauce, bell pepper, and onion. Stir well and cover, simmer over low heat for 20 minutes.
- Stuff zucchini boats with taco meat and top each with one tablespoon of shredded cheddar cheese.
- Place zucchini boats in a baking dish. Cover the dish with foil and bake in a preheated oven for 35 minutes.
- Top with remaining salsa and chopped cilantro. Serve and enjoy.

Nutritional value: Calories: 297 kcal   Fat: 17 g
Carbs: 12 g   Sugar: 3 g   Protein: 30.2 g
Cholesterol: 96 mg

Turkey Spinach Egg Muffins

Preparation Time: 10 minutes
Cooking Time: 20 minutes **Servings:** 3
Ingredients:

- 5 egg whites
- 2 eggs
- ¼ cup cheddar cheese, shredded
- ¼ cup spinach, chopped
- ¼ cup milk
- 3 lean breakfast turkey sausage
- Pepper
- Salt

Directions:

1. Preheat the oven to 350 F. Grease muffin tray cups and set aside.
2. In a pan, brown the turkey sausage links over medium-high heat until sausage is brown from all the sides.
3. Cut sausage in ½-inch pieces and set aside.
4. In a large bowl, whisk together eggs, egg whites, milk, pepper, and salt. Stir in spinach.
5. Pour egg mixture into the prepared muffin tray.
6. Divide sausage and cheese evenly between each muffin cup.
7. Bake in preheated oven for 20 minutes or until muffins are set. Serve warm and enjoy.

Nutritional value: Calories 123 Fat 8 g Carbs 9 g Sugar 6 g Protein 13 g Cholesterol 123 mg

Lean and Green Crockpot Chili

Preparation Time: 5 minutes
Cooking Time: 45 minutes
Servings: 8
Ingredients:

- 1 pound boneless skinless chicken breasts, cut into strips
- ½ cup chopped onion
- 2 teaspoons ground cumin
- 1 teaspoon minced garlic
- ½ teaspoon chili powder
- Salt and pepper to taste
- 1 ½ cups water
- 1 can green enchilada sauce
- ½ cup dried beans, soaked overnight

Directions:

1. Place all ingredients in a pot.
2. Mix all ingredients until combined.
3. Close the lid and change the heat to medium.
4. Bring to a boil and allow to simmer for 45 minutes or until the beans are cooked.
5. Serve with chopped cilantro on top.

Nutritional value:
Calories per serving: 84 kcal
Protein: 13.4g
Carbs: 3.6 g
Fat: 1.7g
Sugar: 0.8g

Sophie Haye

Chapter 7:

Lean and Green Pork Recipes

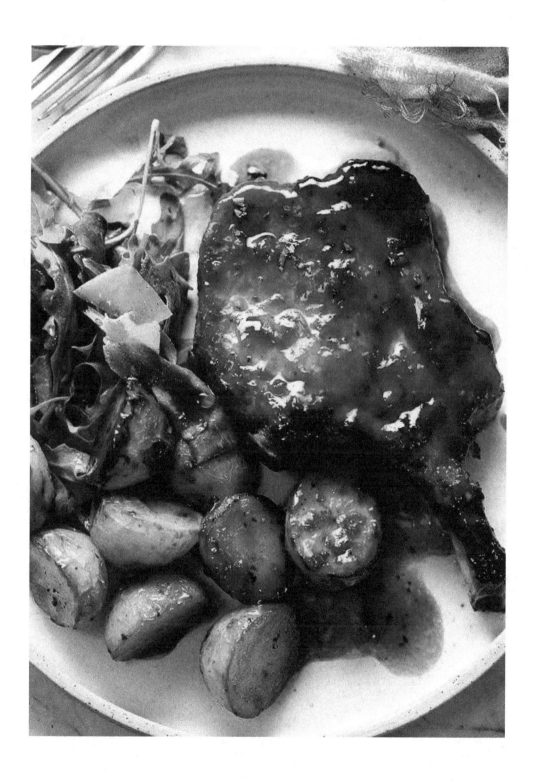

Braised Collard Greens in Peanut Sauce with Pork Tenderloin

Preparation Time: 20 minutes
Cooking Time: 1 hour 12 minutes
Servings: 4
Ingredients:

- 2 cups of chicken stock
- 12 cups of chopped collard greens
- 5 tablespoon of powdered peanut butter
- 3 garlic cloves, crushed
- 1 teaspoon salt
- ½ teaspoon allspice
- ½ teaspoon black pepper
- 2 teaspoon lemon juice
- ¾ teaspoon hot sauce
- 1 ½ pound pork tenderloin

Directions:

1. Get a pot with a tight-fitting lid and combine the collards with the garlic, chicken stock, hot sauce, and half of the pepper and salt. Cook at low heat for about 1 hour or until the collards become tender.
2. Once the collards are tender, stir in the allspice, lemon juice. Add the powdered peanut butter. Keep warm.
3. Season the pork tenderloin with the remaining pepper and salt, and broil in a toaster oven for 10 minutes when you have an internal temperature of 145°F. Make sure to turn the tenderloin every 2 minutes to achieve an even browning all over. After that, you can take away the pork from the oven and allow it to rest for like 5 minutes.
4. Slice the pork and serve.

Nutritional value:
Calories: 320 Fat: 10 g
Carbohydrate: 15 g Protein: 45 g

Oregano Pork Mix

Preparation Time: 5 minutes
Cooking Time: 7 hours and 6 minutes
Servings: 4
Ingredients:

- 2 pounds pork roast
- 7 ounces tomato paste
- 1 yellow onion, chopped
- 1 cup beef stock
- 2 tablespoons ground cumin
- 2 tablespoons olive oil
- 2 tablespoons fresh oregano, chopped
- 1 tablespoon garlic, minced
- ½ cup fresh thyme, chopped

Directions:

1. Heat up a sauté pan with the oil over medium-high heat, add the roast, brown it for 3 minutes on each side and then transfer to your slow cooker.
2. Add the rest of the ingredients, toss a bit, cover and cook on low for 7 hours.
3. Slice the roast, divide it between plates and serve.

Nutritional value:
Calories 623 kcal
Fat 30.1 g
Fiber 6.2 g
Carbs 19.3 g
Protein 69,2 g

Pork and Peppers Chili
Preparation Time: 5 minutes
Cooking Time: 8 hours 5 minutes
Servings: 4
Ingredients:

- 1 red onion, chopped
- 2 pounds pork, ground
- 4 garlic cloves, minced
- 2 red bell peppers, chopped
- 1 celery stalk, chopped
- 25 ounces fresh tomatoes, peeled, crushed
- ¼ cup green chilies, chopped
- 2 tablespoons fresh oregano, chopped
- 2 tablespoons chili powder
- A pinch of salt and black pepper
- A drizzle of olive oil

Directions:

1. Heat up a sauté pan with the oil over medium-high heat and add the onion, garlic and the meat. Mix and brown for 5 minutes then transfer to your slow cooker.
2. Add the rest of the ingredients, toss, cover and cook on low for 8 hours.
3. Divide everything into bowls and serve.

Nutritional value:
Calories 448 kcal
Fat 13 g
Fiber 6.6 g
Carbs 20.2 g
Protein 63 g

Pork Tenderloins and Mushrooms
Preparation Time: 10 minutes
Cooking Time: 25 minutes
Servings: 4
Ingredients:

- on-stick cooking spray
- 1 tablespoon garlic
- 1 tablespoon marjoram
- 1 tablespoon basil
- 1 tablespoon onion
- 1 tablespoon parsley
- 1 ½ pounds pork tenderloin (or beef tenderloin, or chicken breasts)
- 6 cups portobello mushroom caps, cut into chunks
- ½ cups low sodium chicken broth
- 1 tablespoon Stacey Hawkins Garlic Gusto or Garlic & Spring Onion Seasoning (or garlic, salt, black pepper, onion, paprika and parsley)
- Fresh parsley for decorating if desired

Directions:

1. Spray a large skillet with cooking spray.
2. Preheat on stove to medium heat.
3. Place garlic and herbs into the skillet to cook with the cooking spray.
4. Allow the garlic and herbs to cook for 1 minute.
5. Place the pork tenderloin into the pan.
6. Generously season the pork tenderloin with the garlic to taste.
7. Sear the pork for 5 minutes and flip to the other side. Sear the other side for an additional minute.
8. Add the mushrooms, broth, and 2 tablespoons of water into the pan.
9. Cover the pan for 20 minutes.
10. Uncover and let it simmer for an additional 10 minutes till tender.
11. Decorate with marjoram. Serve hot.

Nutritional value:
Calories: 737 kcal
Fat: 62.95 g   Protein: 30.32 g
Carbohydrates: 14.39 g
Calcium: 40 mg
Magnesium: 48 mg
Phosphorus: 443 mg

Juicy Rosemary Pulled Pork
Preparation Time: 10 minutes
Cooking Time: 35 minutes
Servings: 4
Ingredients
- 1 tablespoon olive oil
- 1 teaspoon sea salt
- ½ teaspoon ground black pepper
- 4 boneless center-cut pork chops
- 6-8 cloves garlic, peeled and whole

Directions:
1. Combine the olive oil, salt and pepper in a small bowl. Rub into the pork chops. Refrigerate for 30 minutes.
2. Rub 2 cloves of garlic into the pork chops.
3. Preheat the grill.
4. Grill the pork chops for 6-8 minutes on each side or until done.
5. Chop the remaining cloves of garlic and add them to a bowl with the rosemary, onion, and barbecue sauce. Whisk to blend.
6. Preheat the oven to 325°F.
7. Thinly slice the red onion and place it in a bowl. Add enough balsamic vinegar to cover it and let it marinate for 10 minutes.
8. In the same bowl, add the tomato halves. Sprinkle it with garlic, salt and olive oil. Stir to cover everything evenly.
9. Place the onions in the bottom of a baking dish. Place the pork chops on top and pour over any leftover marinade.
10. Cook covered for 30-35 minutes.
11. To make the sauce, place all the ingredients into a blender and blend until smooth.
12. Serve pork with sauce and lime wedges on the side.

Nutritional value:
Calories: 265 kcal
Phosphorus: 400 mg
Protein: 39.52 g
Magnesium: 48 mg
Fat: 10.02 g
Carbohydrates: 1.98 g
Calcium: 44 mg

Brown Sugar Italian Pork
Preparation Time: 15 minutes
Cooking Time: 6 minutes
Servings: 6
Ingredients:
- 6 boneless pork chops
- ¾ cup white wine
- ½ cup brown sugar
- 3 tablespoons Italian seasoning
- 1 tablespoon olive oil

Directions:
1. Heat the olive oil in your cooker with the lid off, on the "chicken/meat" setting.
2. While that heats up, season pork generously with Italian seasoning and brown sugar.
3. Add pork to the cooker and sear on both sides till it gets golden.
4. Pour in the white wine and seal the lid.
5. Adjust cook time to 6 minutes.
6. When time is up, hit "cancel" and quick-release.
7. Make sure the pork has reached 145°F.
8. Rest for 5 minutes before serving.

Nutritional value:
Total calories: 315 kcal Protein: 23 g
Carbs: 27 g Fat: 13 g   Fiber: 0g

Apricot-Glazed Pork Chops

Preparation Time: 15 minutes
Cooking Time: 6 minutes
Servings: 6
Ingredients:

- 6 boneless pork chops
- ½ cup apricot preserves
- 1 tablespoon balsamic vinegar
- 2 teaspoons olive oil
- Black pepper to taste

Directions:

1. Add oil to your cooker and hit "chicken/meat," leaving the lid off.
2. Sprinkle black pepper on the pork chops.
3. Sear chops in the cooker on both sides till golden.
4. Mix the balsamic and apricot preserves together.
5. Pour over the pork and seal the cooker lid.
6. Adjust cook time to 6 minutes.
7. When time is up, hit "cancel" and quick-release.
8. Test temperature of pork - it should be 145°F.
9. Rest for 5 minutes before serving.

Nutritional value:

Total calories: 296 kcal
Protein: 20g
Carbs: 18g
Fat: 16g
Fiber: 0g

Easy Pork Ribs

Preparation Time: 10 minutes
Cooking Time: 15 minutes
Servings: 6
Ingredients:

- 3 pounds boneless pork ribs
- ½ cup soy sauce
- ¼ cup ketchup
- 2 tablespoons olive oil
- Black pepper to taste

Directions:

1. Pour oil into your pressure cooker and hit "chicken/meat," leaving the lid off.
2. When the oil is hot, add the ribs and sear till golden on both sides.
3. In a bowl, mix black pepper, soy sauce, and ketchup.
4. Pour over the ribs and seal the lid.
5. Adjust cook time to 15 minutes.
6. When the time is up, hit "cancel" and wait 5 minutes before quick-releasing.
7. Make sure pork is at least 145°F before serving.

Nutritional value::

Total calories: 570 kcal
Protein: 65g
Carbs: 0g
Fat: 27g
Fiber: 0g

Pineapple-BBQ Pork
Preparation Time: 10 minutes
Cooking Time: 6 minutes
Servings: 4
Ingredients:
- 4 bone-in pork loin chops
- 8 ounce can undrained crushed pineapple
- 1 cup honey BBQ sauce
- 2 tablespoons chili sauce
- 1 tablespoon olive oil

Directions:
1. Mix the can of pineapple, BBQ sauce, and chili sauce.
2. Turn your pressure cooker to "chicken/meat" and heat.
3. When hot, add the olive oil.
4. When the oil is sizzling, sear pork chops on both sides, 3-4 minutes per side.
5. When brown, pour sauce over the pork and seal the lid.
6. Adjust time to 6 minutes.
7. When time is up, hit "cancel" and wait 5 minutes before quick-releasing.
8. Pork should be cooked to 145°F.
9. Serve with sauce.

Nutritional value:
Total calories: 370 kcal
Protein: 28 g
Carbs: 37 g
Fat: 13g
Fiber: 0 g

Apple-Garlic Pork Loin
Preparation Time: 5 minutes
Cooking Time: 25 minutes
Servings: 12
Ingredients:
- 3 pound boneless pork loin roast
- 12 ounce jar apple jelly
- ⅓ cup water
- 1 tablespoon Herbes de Provence
- 2 teaspoons minced garlic

Directions:
1. Put the pork loin in your cooker. Cut in half if necessary.
2. Mix the garlic, water, and jelly.
3. Pour over the pork.
4. Season with Herbes de Provence.
5. Seal the lid.
6. Hit "chicken/meat" and adjust time to 25 minutes.
7. When time is up, hit "cancel" and wait 10 minutes before quick-releasing.
8. Pork should be served at 145°F. If it's not cooked through yet, hit "chicken/meat" and cook with the lid off until temperature is reached.
9. Rest for 15 minutes before slicing.

Nutritional value:
Total calories: 236 kcal
Protein: 26 g
Carbs: 19 g
Fat: 6 g
Fiber: 0g

Pork with Cranberry-Honey Gravy

Preparation Time: 10 minutes
Cooking Time: 72 minutes **Servings:** 4
Ingredients:

- 2 ½ pounds bone-in pork shoulder
- 15 ounces can whole-berry cranberry sauce
- ¼ cup minced onion
- ¼ cup honey
- Salt to taste

Directions:

1. Add all the ingredients into your pressure cooker and seal the lid.
2. Hit "chicken/meat" and adjust time to 1 hour and 12 minutes.
3. When time is up, hit "cancel" and wait 10 minutes for a natural pressure release.
4. Remove the lid and de-bone.
5. Serve the pork with gravy.

Nutritional value:

Total calories: 707 kcal
Protein: 43g
Carbs: 61g
Fat: 30g
Fiber: 0g

Mexican-Braised Pork with Sweet Potatoes

Preparation Time: 10 minutes
Cooking Time: 25 minutes **Servings:** 4
Ingredients:

- 3 pounds pork loin
- 2 peeled and diced sweet potatoes
- 1 cup tomato salsa
- ½ cup chicken stock
- 1/3 cup Mexican spice blend

Directions:

1. Season the pork all over with the spice blend.
2. Turn your cooker to "chicken/meat" and heat.
3. When hot, sear the pork on both sides. If the meat sticks, pour in a little chicken stock.
4. When the pork is golden, pour in the stock and salsa.
5. Tumble sweet potatoes on one side of the pot and seal the lid.
6. Adjust time to 25 minutes.
7. When the time is up, hit "cancel" and wait 10 minutes before quick-releasing.
8. The pork should be cooked to 145°F, and the potatoes should be tender.
9. Remove the pork and rest 8-10 minutes before serving.

Nutritional value:

Total calories: 513 kcal
Protein: 73 g Carbs: 17 g
Fat: 14 g
Fiber: 1 g

Peach-Mustard Pork Shoulder
Preparation Time: 2 minutes
Cooking Time: 55 minutes
Servings: 8
Ingredients:
- 4 pounds pork shoulder
- 1 cup peach
- 1 cup white wine
- 1/3 cup salt
- 1 tablespoon grainy mustard

Directions:
1. Season the pork well with salt.
2. Mix the mustard and peach, and rub on the pork.
3. Pour wine into the cooker and add the pork.
4. Seal the lid.
5. Hit "chicken/meat" and adjust time to 55 minutes.
6. When time is up, hit "cancel" and wait 10 minutes before quick-releasing.
7. Pork should be cooked to at least 145°F.
8. Move pork to a plate and tent with foil for 15 minutes before slicing and serving.

Nutritional value:
Total calories: 583 kcal Protein: 44g
Carbs: 26g Fat: 32g Fiber: 0g

Pork Cacciatore
Preparation Time: 10 minutes
Cooking Time: 6 hours
Servings: 6
Ingredients:
- 1 ½ lbs pork chops
- 1 teaspoon dried oregano
- 1 cup beef broth
- 3 tablespoon tomato paste
- 14 oz can tomato, diced
- 2 cups mushrooms, sliced
- 1 small onion, diced
- 1 garlic clove, minced
- 2 tablespoon olive oil
- ¼ teaspoon pepper
- ½ teaspoon salt

Directions:
1. Heat oil in a pan over medium heat.
2. Add pork chops in pan and cook until brown on both the sides.
3. Transfer pork chops into the crock pot.
4. Pour remaining ingredients over the pork chops.
5. Cover and cook on low heat for 6 hours.
6. Serve and enjoy.

Nutritional value:
Calories: 440 kcal Fat: 33 g
Carbohydrates: 6 g Sugar: 3 g
Protein: 28 g Cholesterol: 97 mg

Pork with Tomato & Olives

Preparation Time: 10 minutes
Cooking Time: 30 minutes
Servings: 6
Ingredients:

- 6 pork chops, boneless and cut into thick slices
- 1/8 teaspoon ground cinnamon
- 1/2 cup olives, pitted and sliced
- 8 oz can tomato, crushed
- 1/4 cup beef broth
- 2 garlic cloves, chopped
- 1 large onion, sliced
- 1 tablespoon olive oil

Directions:

1. Heat olive oil in a pan over medium heat.
2. Place pork chops in a pan and cook until lightly brown and set aside.
3. Cook onion and garlic in the same pan over medium heat, until onion is softened.
4. Add broth and bring to boil over high heat.
5. Return pork to pan and stir in crushed tomatoes and remaining ingredients.
6. Cover and simmer for 20 minutes.
7. Serve and enjoy.

Nutritional value:

Calories: 321 kcal Fat: 23 g Carbohydrates: 7 g
Sugar: 1 g Protein: 19 g Cholesterol: 70 mg

Tomatillo and Green Chili Pork Stew

Preparation Time: 10 minutes
Cooking Time: 20 minutes
Servings: 4
Ingredients:

- 2 Scallions, chopped
- 2 Cloves of garlic
- 1 lb. Tomatillos, trimmed and chopped
- 8 Large romaine or green lettuce leaves, divided
- 2 Serrano chilies, seeds, and membranes
- ½ Tsp of dried Mexican oregano (or you can use regular oregano)
- 1 ½ lb. of boneless pork loin, to be cut into bite-sized cubes
- ¼ Cup of cilantro, chopped
- ¼ Tablespoon (each) salt and paper
- 1 Jalapeno, seeds and membranes to be removed and thinly sliced
- 1 Cup of sliced radishes
- 4 Lime wedges

Directions:

1. Combine scallions, garlic, tomatillos, four lettuce leaves, serrano chilies, and oregano in a blender. Then puree until smooth.
2. Put pork and tomatillo mixture in a medium pot. 1-inch of puree should cover the pork; if not, add water until it covers it. Season with pepper & salt, and cover it simmers. Simmer for approximately 20 minutes.
3. Now, finely shred the remaining lettuce leaves.
4. When the stew is done cooking, garnish with cilantro, radishes, finely shredded lettuce, sliced jalapenos, and lime wedges.

Nutritional value:

Calories: 370 kcal

Protein: 36g

Carbohydrate: 14g

Fat: 19g

Sweet Potato Bacon Mash
Preparation Time: 10 minutes
Cooking Time: 20 minutes
Servings: 4
Ingredients:
- 3 sweet potatoes, peeled
- 4 oz. bacon, chopped
- 1 cup chicken stock
- 1 tablespoon butter
- 1 teaspoon salt
- 2 ounces Parmesan, grated

Directions:
1. Chop the sweet potato and put it in the pan.
2. Add the chicken stock and close the lid.
3. Boil the vegetables for 15 minutes or until they are soft.
4. After this, drain the chicken stock.
5. Mash the sweet potato with the help of the potato masher. Add grated cheese and butter.
6. Mix up together salt and chopped bacon. Fry the mixture until it is crunchy (10-15 minutes).
7. Add cooked bacon in the mashed sweet potato and mix up with the help of the spoon.
8. It is recommended to serve the meal warm or hot.

Nutritional value:
Calories 304 kcal
Fat 18.1 g
Fiber 2.9 g
Carbs 18.8 g
Protein 17 g

Prosciutto Wrapped Mozzarella Balls
Preparation Time: 10 minutes
Cooking Time: 10 minutes
Servings: 4
Ingredients:
- 8 Mozzarella balls, cherry size
- 4 ounces bacon, sliced
- ¼ teaspoon ground black pepper
- ¾ teaspoon dried rosemary
- 1 teaspoon butter

Directions:
1. Sprinkle the sliced bacon with ground black pepper and dried rosemary.
2. Wrap every Mozzarella ball in the sliced bacon and secure them with toothpicks.
3. Melt butter.
4. Brush wrapped Mozzarella balls with butter.
5. Line the tray with the baking paper and arrange Mozzarella balls in it.
6. Bake the meal for 10 minutes at 365°F.

Nutritional value:
Calories 323 kcal
Fat 26.8 g
Fiber 0.1 g
Carbs 0.6 g
Protein 20.6 g

Prosciutto Spinach Salad

Preparation Time: 5 minutes
Cooking Time: 5 minutes
Servings: 2
Ingredients:

- 2 cups baby spinach
- ⅓ pounds prosciutto
- 1 melon
- 1 avocado
- ¼ cup diced red onions
- Handful of raw unsalted walnuts
- Ground black pepper (optional)

Directions:

1. Put a cup of spinach on each plate.
2. Top with the diced prosciutto, cubes of melon, slices of avocado, a handful of red onion and a few walnuts.
3. Add some ground pepper, if you like.
4. Serve!

Nutritional value:
Calories: 348 kcal
Carbs: 11 g
Fat: 9 g
Protein: 26 g
Fiber: 22 g

Summer Squash Pappardelle with Sausage Ragout

Preparation time: 10 minutes
Cooking time: 10 minutes
Servings: 4
Ingredients:

- 4 Cups summer squash noodles
- 1 ¼ pounds turkey sausage (85-94% lean)
- 2 Cups fresh chopped tomatoes or diced canned tomatoes (no sugar added)
- ½ tablespoon Stacey Hawkins' Viva Italian Seasoning (or basil, oregano, marjoram, onion, and garlic)
- ½ tablespoon Stacey Hawkins' Garlic Gusto Seasoning (or fresh garlic, paprika, parsley, and onion)
- A pinch Stacey Hawkins' Dash of Desperation Seasoning

Directions:

1. Preheat Oven to 400 degrees
2. Slice the squash to the same size as the pasta you are using. Thinner slices cook faster.
3. Boil the noodles in salted water for about 2 minutes.
4. Spread the squash in a thin layer on a baking sheet sprayed with non-stick cooking spray
5. Bake for 10 minutes (total cooking time).
6. Meanwhile, cook the sausages with the seasoning and tomato in a frying pan over medium
7. heat.
8. Drain the noodles and combine it with the sausage ragout.
9. Serve. Note: Top it with grated parmesan if you can tolerate dairy.

Nutritional value:
Calories: 316 kcal
Protein: 36.21 g
Fat: 15.3 g
Carbohydrates: 8.18 g
Calcium: 88 mg
Magnesium: 61 mg

'I Love Bacon'
Preparation Time: 35 minutes
Cooking Time: 90 minutes
Servings: 4
Ingredients:
- 30 slices thick-cut bacon
- 12 ounces steak
- 10 ounces pork sausage
- 4 ounces cheddar cheese, shredded

Directions:
1. Lay out 5 or 6 slices of bacon in a woven pattern and bake at 400°F for 20 minutes until crisp.
2. Combine the steak, bacon and sausage to form a meaty mixture.
3. Lay out the meat in a rectangle of similar size to the bacon strips. Season with salt and pepper.
4. Place the bacon weave on top of the meat mixture.
5. Place the cheese in the center of the bacon.
6. Roll the meat into a tight roll and refrigerate.
7. Make a 7 x 7 bacon weave and roll it over the meat, diagonally.
8. Bake at 400°F for 60 minutes or 165°F internally.
9. Let it rest for 5 minutes before serving.

Nutritional value:
Calories: 190 kcal
Carbs: 17 g
Fat: 15 g
Protein: 39 g
Fiber: 53 g

Garlic Crusted BBQ Baby Back Ribs
Preparation Time: 15 minutes
Cooking Time: 1 hour **Servings:** 2
Ingredients
- 11 ¾ rack baby back ribs
- 2 tablespoon extra-virgin olive oil
- Kosher salt and freshly ground pepper
- 6 garlic cloves
- 12 sprig thyme
- 8 sage leaves with stems
- 2 sprig rosemary

Directions:
1. Preheat the oven to 350°F.
2. Season the ribs with salt and pepper and pinch it all over with a fork. Rub both sides with olive oil and place them in a roasting rack set over a baking sheet. Sprinkle garlic over the meat, and place 4 sage leaves and 4 rosemary leaves on top of the meat.
3. Bake the ribs for 30 minutes. Reduce the oven temperature to 300°F and bake the ribs for 25 minutes.
4. Place 4 more sage leaves and 4 rosemary leaves on top of the meat. Bake for another 30 minutes.
5. Place 1 cup of barbecue sauce in a bowl. Scrape all the sauce from the roaster.
6. Return the ribs to the pan and brush the meat with the sauce. Bake for 15 additional minutes.
7. Scrape again, the sauce from the roaster and spread it over the meat.
8. Remove the meat from the oven and serve with more sauce.

Nutritional value:
Calories: 19863 kcal
Protein: 1754.29 g Fat: 1401.07 g
Carbohydrates: 82.05 g Calcium: 1903 mg
Magnesium: 2170 mg Phosphorus: 12527 mg

Lightened-Up Bangers & Mash

Preparation Time: 3 minutes
Cooking Time: 20 minutes
Servings: 6
Ingredients:

- 6 x 4 ounce pork sausages (raw)
- 3 pounds peeled and diced butternut squash
- 1 cup chicken broth
- 1 chopped onion
- 1 tablespoon Dijon mustard

Directions:

1. Poke the sausages a few times.
2. Put squash in the pot and pour in the chicken broth.
3. Add in Dijon.
4. Add it to the slow cooker and pile in sausages with onion on top.
5. Seal the lid.
6. Hit "chicken/meat" and adjust time to 20 minutes.
7. When time is up, hit "cancel" and quick-release.
8. Sausage should be cooked to 145°F, while the squash is tender.
9. Serve!

Nutritional value:

Total calories: 506 kcal
Protein: 19 g zCarbs: 29 g
Fat: 36 g
Fiber: 5 g

Easy BBQ Meatballs

Preparation Time: 5 minutes
Cooking Time: 20 minutes
Servings: 1
Ingredients:

- Turkey Meatballs: Trader Joes (5), Jennie-O Homestyle (6) or Butterball Italian Style (10)
- ¼ cup Guy's Smokey Garlic BBQ Sauce
- 1 teaspoon Low sodium soy sauce

Directions:

1. Bake meatballs according to the package. (Trader Joes is 20 minutes at 350° Fahrenheit.)
2. Whisk the soy and BBQ sauce in a small bowl and pour over meatballs.

Nutritional value:

Calories: 2281 kcal
Protein: 90.03 g
Fat: 176.16 g
Carbohydrates: 90.59 g

Coq au Vin

Preparation Time: 10 minutes.
Cooking Time: 40 minutes.
Servings: 2.

Ingredients

- 450 grams (1-pound) button mushrooms.
- 100 grams (3½ ounces) streaky bacon, chopped.
- 16 chicken thighs, skin removed.
- 3 cloves of garlic, crushed.
- 3 tablespoon of fresh parsley, chopped.
- 3 carrots, chopped.
- 2 red onions, chopped.
- 2 tablespoons of plain flour.
- 2 tablespoons of olive oil.
- 750 milliliters (1¼ pints) red wine.
- 1 bouquet garni.

Directions

1. Place the flour on a large plate and coat the chicken in it.
2. Heat the olive oil in a large saucepan, add the chicken and brown it, before setting aside.
3. Fry the bacon in the pan then add the onion and cook for 5 minutes.
4. Pour in the red wine and add the chicken, carrots, bouquet garni, and garlic.
5. Transfer it to a large ovenproof dish.
6. Cook in the oven at 180°C/360°F for 1 hour.
7. Remove the bouquet garni and skim off any excess fat, if necessary.
8. Add in the mushrooms and cook for 15 minutes.
9. Stir in the parsley just before serving.

Nutrition

- Calories: 322 kcal. Fat: 6 g.
- Fiber: 8 g. Carbs: 5 g.

Chapter 8:

Lean and Green Beef Recipes

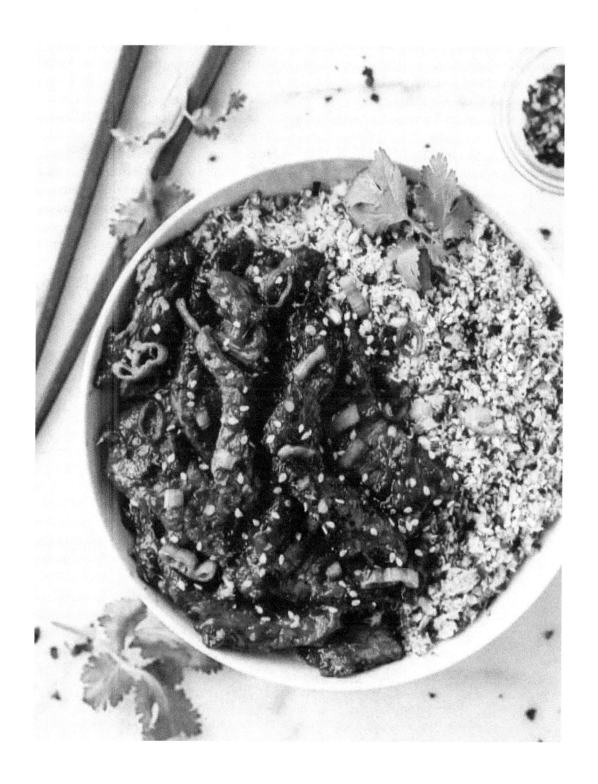

Lean and Green "Macaroni"

Preparation Time: 5 minutes
Cooking Time: 10 minutes
Servings: 4
Ingredients:

- 2tablespoons yellow onion, diced
- 5 ounces 95-97% lean ground beef
- 2tablespoons light thousand island dressing
- ⅛ teaspoon apple cider vinegar
- ⅛ teaspoon onion powder
- 3 cups Romaine lettuce, shredded
- 2tablespoons low-fat cheddar cheese, shredded
- 1-ounce dill pickle slices
- 1teaspoon sesame seeds

Directions:

1. Pour three tablespoons of water into a pan and heat over a medium-low flame. Sauté the onions for 30 seconds before adding the beef. Sauté the meat for 4 minutes while stirring constantly.
2. Add in the thousand island dressing, apple cider vinegar, and onion powder. Close the lid and keep on cooking for 5 minutes. Remove the lid and allow it to simmer until the sauce thickens. Turn off the heat and allow the beef to rest and cool.
3. Place the lettuce at the bottom and pour in the beef—layer with cheddar cheese and pickles in a bowl. Sprinkle with sesame on top.

Nutritional value:
Calories per serving:119kcal
Protein: 10.8g
Carbs: 4.4g Fat: 2.1g
Sugar: 2.5g

Lean and Green Broccoli Taco

Preparation Time: 5 minutes
Cooking Time: 15 minutes
Servings: 4
Ingredients:

- 4 ounces 95-97% lean ground beef
- ¼ cup Roma tomatoes, chopped
- ¼ teaspoon garlic powder
- ¼ teaspoon onion powder
- 1 ¼ cup broccoli, cut into bite-sized pieces
- A pinch of red pepper flakes
- 1-ounce low-sodium cheddar cheese, shredded

Directions:

1. Place three tablespoons of water in a pan and heat over medium flame. Sauté the beef and tomatoes for 5 minutes until the tomatoes are wilted. Add in the garlic and onion powder, then stir for another 3 minutes.
2. Add the broccoli and close the lid. Cook for another 5 minutes.
3. Garnish with red pepper flakes and cheddar cheese on top.

Nutritional value:
Calories per serving:97
Protein:9.9 g
Carbs: 2.6g
Fat: 1.7g
Sugar:0.9 g

Cumin-Lime Steak

Preparation Time: 30 minutes
Cooking Time: 30 minutes **Servings:** 4
Ingredients:

- Seaweed
- 20 Once. Steak with lean rib-eye
- 6 Tops Broccoli
- 1 Pack quick bovine soup (prepared as directed) or 1/2 cup beef broth
- ¼ tablespoon lime juice
- 1 ½ spoonfuls ground cumin
- 1 ½ spoonfuls ground coriander
- 2 Large, finely chopped cloves garlic
- 3 Pounds olive oil

Directions:

1. Mix all marinade ingredients (except oil) together in a blender.
2. Add oil to mixer with motor working slowly.
3. Refrigerate and cover until ready to use. Pour 1 cup of marinade over steaks in a glass dish, covering with all sides.
4. Cover and leave to cool for 6 hours (or overnight).
5. Grill over medium-sized coals, turning regularly and clean with ½ cup marinade left over.
6. Steam broccoli on the side and serve.

Nutritional value:
Fats: 0.7 g
Sodium: 6.1 mg
Carbohydrates: 4.5 g

Cumin Bistec Tacos

Preparation Time: 5 minutes
Cooking Time: 25 minutes
Servings: 4
Ingredients:

- 1 cup fresh cilantro, to be chopped
- 8 radishes must be thinly sliced
- 16 Jicama "tortillas" (large, thinly sliced jicama)
- ¼ teaspoon pepper
- ¼ teaspoon salt
- ½ tablespoon cumin
- 2 tablespoons lime juice
- 2 pounds top the round roast should be chopped or minced.

Directions:

1. Combine the beef with cumin, lime juice, pepper, and salt
2. Get a nonstick skillet and grease it lightly before placing on high heat, then add the beef. Allow the beef to become brown on one side before you stir it and after that, sauté the meat until it is evenly cooked through.
3. Serve the beef in Jicama "tortillas" with cilantro and sliced radishes.

Nutritional value:
Calories: 310 kcal
Protein: 48 g
Carbohydrate: 8 g
Fat: 10 g

Balsamic Beef and Mushrooms Mix
Preparation Time: 5 minutes
Cooking Time: 8 hours
Servings: 4
Ingredients:
- 2 pounds beef, cut into strips
- ¼ cup balsamic vinegar
- 2 cups beef stock
- 1 tablespoon ginger, grated
- ½ lemon, juiced
- 1 cup brown mushrooms, sliced
- A pinch of salt and black pepper
- 1 teaspoon ground cinnamon

Directions:
1. Mix all the ingredients in your slow cooker, cover and cook on low for 8 hours.
2. Divide everything between plates and serve.

Nutritional value:
Calories 446 kcal
Fat 14 g
Fiber 0.6 g
Carbs 2.9 g
Protein 70,8 g

Simple Beef Roast
Preparation Time: 10 minutes
Cooking Time: 8 hours
Servings: 8
Ingredients:
- 5 pounds beef roast
- 2 tablespoons Italian seasoning
- 1 cup beef stock
- 1 tablespoon sweet paprika
- 3 tablespoons olive oil

Directions:
1. In your slow cooker, mix all the ingredients, cover and cook on low for 8 hours.
2. Carve the roast, divide it between plates and serve.

Nutritional value:
Calories 587 kcal
Fat 24.1 g
Fiber 0.3 g
Carbs 0.9 g
Protein 86.5 g

Taco Bowls with Cauliflower Rice
Preparation time: 10 minutes
Cooking time: 20 minutes **Servings:** 4
Ingredients:
For the taco meat:
- 1 teaspoon olive oil
- 1 pound ground beef
- 1 teaspoon paprika
- 1 teaspoon pepper
- 1 teaspoon chili powder
- 1 teaspoon garlic powder
- ½ teaspoon salt - 1 teaspoon onion powder - 1 teaspoon cumin

For cauliflower rice:
- 1 pound cauliflower rice
- 1 teaspoon olive oil
- ¼ cup lemon juice
- 1 teaspoon lemon zest
- 2 tablespoons cilantro fresh, chopped

For the toppings:
- 1 cup avocado sliced
- 1 cup FAGE Total 0% Yogurt
- 1 cup shredded cheddar cheese
- 1 cup tomatoes, halved
- 1 cup olives, halved

Directions:
1. Make the cauliflower rice
2. Place the cauliflower in a food processor and press star until it's the consistency of rice.
3. Add salt to taste and press start for another 5 seconds.
4. Heat the olive oil in a pan over medium heat. Add the cauliflower rice to the pan, stir until all of the cauliflower rice is coated.
5. Cook for 5 minutes with the lid on. Remove the lid and add the lemon juice, stir until it reaches the desired consistency.
6. Stir in the lemon zest and cilantro. Set aside.
   For the taco meat:
7. Heat the olive oil in a large pan over medium heat. Add the garlic and onion, stir for a few minutes.
8. Add the ground beef, salt, pepper, chili powder, garlic powder, paprika, cumin, and onion powder. Cook until the beef is browned.
9. Remove from heat and drain the fat from the pan.
   For the tacos:
10. In a large bowl, toss together the ingredients in the toppings list.
11. Set aside.
12. Place ¼ cup of cauliflower rice into each taco.
13. Top with ¼ cup of the beef mixture and 1 tablespoon of cheese.
14. Place in the microwave for 5-10 seconds, or in the oven for 2-3 minutes, until the cheese is melted.
15. Add the toppings and enjoy.

Nutritional value: Calories: 462 kcal Protein: 37.31 g Fat: 27.11 g Carbohydrates: 20.18 g Calcium: 197 mg Magnesium: 75 mg

Tender Beef Stew with Rosemary
Preparation Time: 20 minutes
Cooking Time: 2 hours
Servings: 8
Ingredients
- 4 slices bacon, cut into thin strips
- 4 pounds beef chuck roast pieces after trimming - cut into 1 ½ to 2 inch pieces
- ½ teaspoon kosher salt
- ½ teaspoon black pepper
- 1 ½ cups onion chopped
- 2 cups pearl onions fresh, peeled or frozen
- 2 ½ cups carrot pieces peeled and cut into 1 - 1 ½ inch pieces
- 1 tablespoon oil
- ¾ cloves garlic
- 2 sprigs fresh rosemary
- 4 sprigs fresh thyme
- 2 bay leaves dried
- 2 cups low-sodium beef broth
- 2 tablespoons soy sauce
- 2-3 tablespoons butter, softened
- 2-3 tablespoons flour

- 2 tablespoons fresh flat leaf parsley, chopped (optional)

Directions:

1. Place the meat in a large mixing bowl. Sprinkle it with salt and pepper.
2. In a medium-sized sauté pan put the oil, add the bacon strips. Cook over medium heat for about 2-3 minutes.
3. Add the onion, carrot, pearl onions (fresh or frozen), garlic cloves and rosemary springs. Cook for 4-5 minutes until the vegetables start to soften.
4. Add the vegetables and bacon to the meat mixture.
5. Add the thyme, bay leaves and broth.
6. Refrigerate until ready to cook the stew. This can be done a day ahead.
7. After refrigerating the stew, let the stew come to room temperature.
8. Heat the oven to 350 °F.
9. Grease a large baking pan (if needed) and put the meat and vegetables into it.
10. Cover the meat and vegetables with the sauce. Cook for about 90-120 minutes until the meat starts to get tender.
11. Take the meat out of the baking pan and place on a platter or in a large bowl using 2 forks to shred the meat in the pot.
12. Place the meat back in the pot mixture. Add the soy sauce and the butter and give it a stir.
13. Reduce the heat to medium-low. If the stew starts to get very thick and dry, add a little more broth and stir.
14. Mix the 2 tablespoons of flour with ½ cup of water until a very thin paste forms. Stir in the stew while whisking regularly. Add a little extra water if the stew gets too dry. Add the salt and mustard and mix well.
15. Add the parsley to the stew.Serve and enjoy it!

Nutritional value: Calories: 474 kcal Protein: 51.48 g Fat: 22.46 Carbohydrates: 18.46 g Calcium: 85 mg Magnesium: 64 mg Phosphorus: 520 mg

Sesame Beef and Vegetable Stir-fry
Preparation Time: 5 minutes
Cooking Time: 30 minutes **Servings:** 4
Ingredients:

- 1 pound lean top sirloin beef, cut into strips
- 1 bunch asparagus, bottoms cut off and stalks halved
- 1 large handful of green beans, stemmed and cut in half
- 2 onions, diced
- 1 cup vegetable stock
- 2 tablespoons sesame seeds
- 3 teaspoons basil
- 2 tablespoons grapeseed oil
- 2 cups cooked brown rice

Directions:

1. On high heat, warm the grapeseed oil in a frying pan and cook the beef until brown. Remove from the pan.
2. Put the vegetable stock in the pan and heat until boiling. Add the asparagus, green beans, and onions and cook until tender.
3. Add the beef, sesame seeds, basil, and brown rice and cook until everything has absorbed the vegetable stock.
4. Serve warm and enjoy!

Nutritional value:

Calories: 234 kcal

Fat: 5g

Carbs: 8g

Protein: 44g

Cashew Thai Beef Stir-Fry

Preparation Time: 5 minutes
Cooking Time: 30 minutes
Servings: 4
Ingredients:

- 2 garlic cloves, crushed
- 5 tablespoons lemon juice
- 1 tablespoon, rice wine vinegar
- ½ teaspoon cayenne pepper
- 2 teaspoons soy sauce
- 2 sirloin steaks, either New York strip or top sirloin, about 1 pound each, cut into large strips
- 2 tablespoons sesame oil
- 2 onions, diced
- 2 organic bell peppers, sliced into thin strips
- 1 cup broccoli, chopped into florets
- ½ cup cashews
- 2 tablespoons grapeseed oil

Directions:

1. Mix the garlic, lemon juice, rice wine vinegar, cayenne pepper, and soy sauce. Set aside.
2. Brush the beef with the sesame oil. On high heat, add the grapeseed oil in the pan and when it is hot, fry the beef in two batches until it is browned and cooked. Remove from the pan and set aside.
3. Sauté onions until they are tender. Add the peppers and broccoli and cook for 4 minutes. Add cashews and cook for 2 minutes.
4. Put the beef back in and cook until warm. Serve with rice if you desire.

Nutritional value:
Calories: 253 kcal
Fat: 27g Carbs: 36g Protein: 12g

Western Beef Casserole

Preparation Time: 5 minutes **Cooking Time:** 30 minutes **Servings:** 4
Ingredients:

- 1 ½ pounds of ground beef, lean
- 1 cup spanish onion, chopped
- 2 cups corn, canned or frozen
- 2 cups kidney beans
- ½ teaspoon chili powder
- 1 ½ cups tomato soup
- ¼ cup milk - 1 cup cheddar cheese, grated

Directions:

To Prepare for Freezing:
In a frying pan, cook the ground beef until it is brown. Drain excess grease. Place the meat into a large bowl. Wash and chop the onion. Add to the ground beef. Drain the corn and add to the ground beef. Toss until the ingredients are well blended. Drain and wash the kidney beans. Add to the ground beef and mix. Make sure the ingredients are well blended to prevent clumps of beans. In a separate bowl, whisk together the tomato soup and milk. Add in the chili powder and mix with the tomato soup. Pour the soup mixture over the ground beef mixture. Mix. Once it is mixed, carefully spoon the mixture into a large freezer bag. Seal. Shred the cheddar cheese, and place into a small freezer bag. Place the meat freezer bag and the cheese freezer bag into a larger freezer bag. Seal and label the freezer bag with the name of the dish, the date you prepped the meal, the cooking time, and the heat setting. Freeze.

o To Slow Cook:
Remove the ingredients from the freezer. Place the cheese in the fridge to use later. Pour the meat mixture into the slow cooker. Set the slow cooker to low heat and cook for 3 hours. After 3 hours, remove the cheese from the freezer bag and sprinkle on top of the ground beef mixture. Stir until the cheese is dispersed evenly throughout the mixture. Put the lid on and continue cooking for 1 hour. Serve warm with a nice biscuit.

Nutritional value: Calories: 187 kcal Fat: 13g Carbs: 12g Protein: 39g

Crockpot Meatloaf
Preparation Time: 5 minutes
Cooking Time: 30 minutes
Servings: 6
Ingredients:
- 1 ½ pounds of ground beef, lean
- ¾ cup breadcrumbs
- ½ cup milk
- 1 packages of dry onion soup mix
- 2 eggs
- 1 cups ketchup
- 1 teaspoon Worcestershire sauce
- ½ cup brown sugar
- ¼ teaspoon ginger, ground
- ¼ teaspoon black pepper
- 1 teaspoon salt
- Non-stick cooking spray

Directions:
To Prepare for Freezing:
1. In a large bowl, mix together the ground beef, breadcrumbs, and onion soup mix.
2. Add in the salt and pepper.
3. Add in the ginger.
4. Slowly pour in the milk, mixing the ground beef mixture as you do.
5. Finally, add the eggs and mix thoroughly.
6. Form the ground beef into a loaf, and place into a large freezer bag. (Optional: you can flatten the ground beef before freezing to save room. When you are ready to cook it, defrost completely and form into a loaf before cooking).
7. In a small bowl, stir together the ketchup and Worcestershire sauce.
8. Add in the brown sugar, and mix until the sugar is dissolved. Pour into a small freezer bag and seal.
9. Place all of the ingredient bags into a large freezer bag.
10. Seal and label the freezer bag with the name of the dish, the date you prepped the meal, the cooking time, and the heat setting.
11. Freeze.
To Slow Cook:
12. Cover the slow cooker with tinfoil.
13. Spray with non-stick cooking spray.
14. Remove the meatloaf from the freezer, and place it in the center of the slow cooker.
15. Place the ketchup bag into the fridge so it can defrost by the end of the day.
16. Cook on low heat for 6 hours.
17. Once it is cooked, remove the ketchup bag, and spread the ketchup onto the meatloaf.
18. Cook for an additional 15 to 20 minutes, and then remove by carefully lifting the tinfoil out of the slow cooker.
19. Serve warm with potatoes or other side dishes.
Nutritional value: Calories: 456 kcal   Fat: 33g   Carbs: 2g   Protein: 19g

Provençal Beef Daube
Preparation Time: 5 minutes
Cooking Time: 30 minutes
Servings: 6
Ingredients:
- 2 pounds boneless chuck roast
- 2 teaspoons olive oil
- 2 cups carrots, chopped
- 1 ½ cups onion, chopped
- 1 tablespoon tomato paste
- 1 teaspoon thyme
- 1 teaspoon rosemary
- 12 garlic cloves
- 1 cup wine
- 1 ¼ teaspoons salt
- ½ teaspoon ground pepper
- 1 ¾ cup diced tomatoes
- ½ cup beef broth
- 1 bay leaf

Directions:
To Prepare for Freezing:
1. Place a skillet on the stove, and add the oil. Set the temperature to low.
2. Cut the beef into 1-inch cubes.
3. Mince the garlic, and place in the hot oil.
4. Cook for about 5 minutes, or until you have a rich, fragrant garlic smell.
5. Remove the garlic with a slotted spoon, set aside.

6. Add the beef, and increase the temperature to medium high.
7. Sprinkle on ½ teaspoon of salt and a ¼ teaspoon of pepper.
8. Cook for about 5 minutes or until the beef is brown on all sides.
9. Remove the beef from the pan, and add it to the garlic.
10. Pour in the wine, and bring to a boil. Make sure you scrape the pan to remove any brown bits that are sticking to the pan.
11. Once it is boiling, stir in the garlic and beef.
12. Add the remaining salt and pepper.
13. Wash, peel, and chop the carrots and onion. Add to the beef mixture.
14. Stir in the beef broth and tomato paste.
15. Add the diced tomatoes.
16. Add in the rosemary and thyme.
17. Bring to boil, then remove from heat.
18. Cool completely before pouring the mixture into a freezer bag.
19. Seal and label the larger bag with the date you prepped the meal as well as the cooking time and heat setting.
20. Freeze.

To Slow Cook:

21. Remove from the freezer, and run the freezer bag under hot water.
22. When a small amount of juice forms, empty the bag into a slow cooker.
23. Add the bay leaf. Set the slow cooker to low, and cook for 5 hours or until the beef is tender. Remove the bay leaf, and discard. Serve warm on its own or over a bed of egg noodles.

Nutritional value: Calories: 165 kcal   Fat: 23g Carbs: 15g Protein: 14g

Pan-Seared Beef Tips and Mushrooms

Preparation Time: 10 minutes
Cooking Time: 25 minutes
Servings: 4
Ingredients:

- 16 ounces lean beef cut into 1 chunk (London broil, filet, strip steak, etc.)
- ½ tablespoon salt
- ½ tablespoon pepper
- ½ tablespoon garlic
- nonstick cooking spray
- 4 cups mushrooms (either small, whole mushrooms or larger ones cut into quarters)
- 1 cup low sodium beef broth
- 1 ½ teaspoons fresh garlic
- 1 ½ teaspoons parsley
- 1 ½ teaspoons onion

Directions:

1. Sprinkle beef with salt, pepper, and garlic.
2. Coat a large skillet with nonstick cooking spray. Heat over medium-high heat and add beef. Cook for about 8-10 minutes, stirring frequently or until beef is browned on all sides and no pink remains.
3. Add mushrooms to the skillet. Pour the beef broth and boil. Cover and cook over low heat for 15 minutes.
4. While beef simmers in mushroom sauce, combine garlic, parsley, and onion in a food processor fitted with a steel blade. Pulse a few times until minced.
5. Add garlic mixture to the beef and mushrooms and simmer covered for 10 minutes more.
6. Place in serving bowls and top with parsley. As an alternative, if desired, top with gouda cheese.

Nutritional value:

Calories: 379 kcal

Protein: 42.49 g Calcium: 66 mg Fat: 12.44 g
Carbohydrates: 25.55 g

Lean and Green Steak Machine

Preparation Time: 5 minutes
Cooking Time: 10 minutes
Servings: 3
Ingredients:

- ½ teaspoon extra virgin olive oil
- 2 ounces Sirloin steak, 98% lean
- Salt and pepper to taste
- 1 zucchini, cut into long thin strips
- 1 onion, chopped
- 6 ounces asparagus, blanched
- 4 ounces peas, blanched

Directions:

1. Heat olive oil in a skillet. If desired, you may season the steak with salt and pepper to taste.
2. Place in the skillet and sear the steak for 5 minutes on each side. Let the meat rest for five minutes before cutting it into strips.
3. Place the remaining ingredients in a bowl and season with salt and pepper to taste
4. Top with steak strips, then mix to combine all ingredients.

Nutritional value:
Calories per serving:174 kcal
Protein: 4.2g
Carbs: 10.3g
Fat: 4.1g
Sugar: 2.1g

Garlic Crusted Flank Steak with Roasted Tomato Relish

Preparation Time: 5 minutes and 1 hour refrigerate **Cooking Time:** 25 minutes**Servings:** 6

Ingredients

For the steak
- 2 tablespoons fresh thyme, chopped
- 2 tablespoons fresh rosemary, chopped
- 1 tablespoon fresh tarragon, chopped
- 2 garlic cloves, minced
- 2 teaspoons salt
- 1 ½ teaspoons ground black pepper
- 2 or 1 ½ pound flank steaks
- 1 tablespoon olive oil
Tomatoes
- 2 cups halved cherry tomatoes

- 1 cup fresh Italian parsley, chopped
- ¼ cup coarsely chopped pitted Kalamata olives or other brine-cured black olives
- ¼ cup coarsely chopped pitted brine-cured green olives
- ¼ cup fresh basil, chopped
- ¼ cup extra-virgin olive oil
- 2 tablespoons sherry wine vinegar

Directions:

Preheat the oven to 375°F.To make the tomatoes, in a bowl, toss together the tomatoes, herbs, olives, and basil with the vinegar and oil; season to taste with salt and pepper. In a food processor, process the tomatoes until smooth. Put in the herb mixture from the steak list, along with the garlic, salt, and pepper until the mixture is chopped finely and the herbs have disappeared. With the motor running, drizzle in the olive oil. The relish can be made a day in advance, covered, and refrigerated. On a flat surface, lay the steaks out side by side. Spoon a third of the relish over the steaks and spread it over the meat with a spatula, being careful not to tear the meat. Sprinkle the herb-garlic mixture and roll up the steaks lengthwise. Place them in a baking dish and drizzle with the olive oil. Let it rest at room temperature for 30 minutes. Roast the steaks for 10 minutes. Turn them and continue roasting until medium rare (135 °F) or medium (140°F), about 10 more minutes. The steaks can rest up to 10 minutes before slicing.

1. Cut the steak rolls across grain into 1 ½ inch-thick slices.
2. Serve the steak between the tomato slices.

Nutritional value:
Calories: 2236 kcal

Protein: 334.68 g	Fat: 84.92 g
Carbohydrates: 10.36 g	Calcium: 372 mg
Magnesium: 359 mg mg	Phosphorus: 3165

Mediterranean London Broil

Preparation time: 1 hour
Cooking time: 10 minutes **Servings:** 6
Ingredients:

- 2-3 ounces top or bottom round steak
- 1 tablespoon kosher or sea salt
- 1 tablespoon minced garlic
- 2 tablespoons fresh oregano, chopped
- 1 tablespoon parsley, chopped
- 2 teaspoons ground cumin
- 1 teaspoon cinnamon
- 1 teaspoon black pepper
- 1 teaspoon ground sumac (can be substituted with lemon juice)
- 2-3 tablespoons olive oil

Directions:

1. Rub all of the spices, salt, and herbs onto both sides of the steak.
2. Put on a plate and set aside.
3. Heat the olive oil in a large frying pan until it gets very hot.
4. Add the steak and sear the meat until all sides are browned, about 5 minutes per side.
5. Reduce the heat, cover it, and let it simmer for about 10 minutes or until the meat is fork-tender.
6. Let the meat rest for 5 minutes and serve.
7. This goes very well with roasted red potatoes and sauteed veggies.

Note: If you don't want to cook your meat in olive oil, I advise adding an additional tablespoon of olive oil after the meat has seared and is ready to be cooked.

Nutritional value:

Calories: 301 kcal Magnesium: 50 mg Protein: 42.16 g Fat: 13.06 g Carbohydrates: 1.48 gCalcium: 27 mg

Chapter 9:

Lean and Green Veggie Recipes

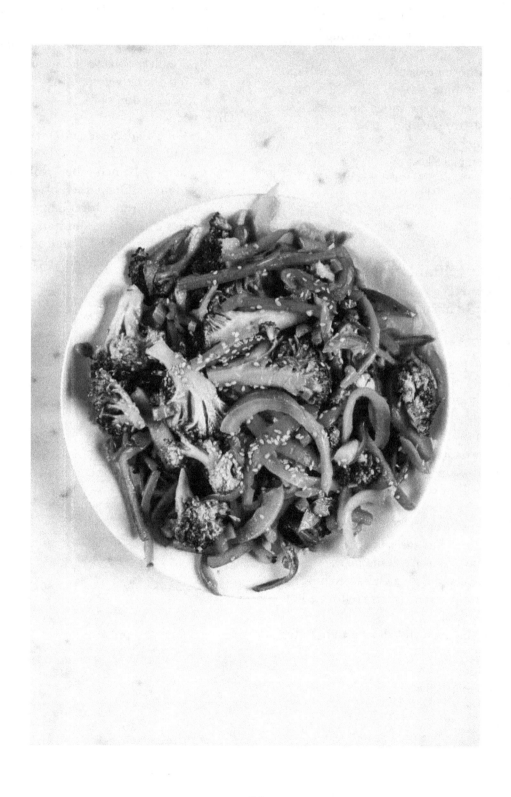

Lean and Green Cauliflower Salad
Preparation Time: 5 minutes
Cooking Time: 3 minutes
Servings: 2
Ingredients:

- 1 cup cauliflower florets
- ¼ cup apple cider vinegar
- One tablespoon Tuscan seasoning

Directions:

1. Add all the ingredients into a bowl and toss to combine.
2. Allow resting in the fridge for at least 30 minutes before serving.

Nutritional value:
Calories per serving: 41 kcal
Protein: 1.3g
Carbs: 8.7g
Fat: 0.1g
Sugar: 2g

Vegetarian Zucchini Lasagna
Preparation Time: 5 minutes
Cooking Time: 10 minutes
Servings: 6
Ingredients:

- One ¼ pounds zucchini, sliced into lasagna
- ¼ cup chopped fresh spinach
- 1 ½ cup sugar-free and low-sodium marinara sauce
- ⅔ cup mozzarella cheese, shredded
- 1 cup part-skim ricotta cheese
- Fresh basil for garnish

Directions:

1. Preheat the oven to 375°F for 5 minutes.
2. Place the zucchini slices in a dish and layer with the spinach, marinara sauce, mozzarella, and ricotta cheese. Repeat the process until several layers are formed.
3. Top with basil.
4. Put it in the oven and allow it to bake for 10 minutes.

Nutritional value:
Calories per serving: 128 kcal
Protein: 12.2g
Carbs: 10.7g Fat: 2.6g
Sugar: 2.1g

Cauliflower with Kale Pesto
Preparation Time: 5 minutes
Cooking Time: 2 minutes
Servings: 6
Ingredients:

- 3 cups cauliflower, cut into florets
- 3 cups raw kale, stems removed
- 2 cups fresh basil
- 2 tablespoons extra virgin olive oil
- 3 tablespoons lemon juice
- 3 garlic cloves
- ¼ teaspoon salt

Directions:

1. Put an adequate amount of water in the pan and bring to a boil over medium flame. Blanch the cauliflower for 2 minutes. Drain, then place it in a bowl of ice-cold water for 5 minutes. Drain again.
2. In a blender, add the rest of the ingredients. Blend until smooth.
3. Pour the pesto over the cooked cauliflower.

Nutritional value:
Calories per serving: 41kcal
Protein: 1.8g
Carbs: 5g Fat: 5.3g
Sugar: 1.4g

Lean and Green Broccoli Alfredo
Preparation Time: 5 minutes
Cooking Time: 2 minutes
Servings: 5
Ingredients:
- 2 heads of broccoli, cut into florets
- 2 tablespoons lemon juice, freshly squeezed
- ½ cup cashew, soaked for 2 hours in water then drained
- 2 tablespoons white miso, low sodium
- 2 teaspoon Dijon mustard
- Freshly ground black pepper

Directions:
1. Boil water in a pot using a medium flame. Blanch the broccoli for 2 minutes, then place it in a bowl of iced water. Drain.
2. In a food processor, place the remaining ingredients and blend until smooth.
3. Pour the alfredo sauce over the broccoli. Mix to get it covered with the sauce.

Nutritional value:
Calories per serving: 359 kcal
Protein: 10.6g
Carbs: 50.2 g
Fat: 8.4g
Sugar: 2.4g

Pesto Zucchini Noodles
Preparation Time: 15 minutes
Cooking Time: minutes 15 minutes
Servings: 4
Ingredients:
- 4 zucchini, spiralized
- 1 tbsp. avocado oil
- 2 garlic cloves, chopped
- 2/3 cup olive oil
- 1/3 cup parmesan cheese, grated
- 2 cups fresh basil
- 1/3 cup almonds
- 1/8 tsp black pepper
- ¾ tsp sea salt

Directions:
1. Add zucchini noodles into a colander and sprinkle with ¼ teaspoon of salt. Cover and let sit for 30 minutes. Drain zucchini noodles well and pat dry.
2. Preheat the oven to 400 F.
3. Place almonds on a parchment-lined baking sheet and bake for 6-8 minutes.
4. Transfer toasted almonds into the food processor and process until coarse.
5. Add olive oil, cheese, basil, garlic, pepper, and remaining salt in a food processor with almonds and process until pesto texture.
6. Heat avocado oil in a large pan over medium-high heat.
7. Add zucchini noodles and cook for 4-5 minutes.
8. Pour pesto over zucchini noodles, mix well and cook for 1 minute.
9. Serve immediately with baked salmon.

Nutritional value:
Calories: 525 Fat 44 g Carbs 3 g Sugar 8 g
Protein 16 g Cholesterol 30 mg

Parmesan Zucchini

Preparation Time: 15 minutes
Cooking Time: 15 minutes
Servings: 4
Ingredients:

- 4 zucchini, quartered lengthwise
- 2 tablespoon fresh parsley, chopped
- 2 tablespoon olive oil
- ¼ teaspoon garlic powder
- ½ teaspoon dried basil
- ½ teaspoon dried oregano
- ½ teaspoon dried thyme
- ½ cup parmesan cheese, grated
- Pepper
- Salt

Directions:

1. Preheat the oven to 350 F. Cover a baking sheet with parchment paper and set aside.
2. In a small bowl, mix together the parmesan cheese, garlic powder, basil, oregano, thyme, pepper, and salt.
3. Arrange the zucchini onto the prepared baking sheet and drizzle with oil and sprinkle with parmesan cheese mixture.
4. Bake in a preheated oven for 15 minutes then grill for 2 minutes or until lightly golden brown.
5. Garnish with parsley and serve immediately.

Nutritional value:
Calories: 244 kcal
Fat: 14 g   Carbs: 7 g   Sugar: 5 g   Protein: 15 g
Cholesterol: 30 mg

Tomato Cucumber Avocado Salad

Preparation Time: 15 minutes
Cooking Time: 0 minutes
Servings: 4
Ingredients:

- 12 ounces cherry tomatoes, cut in half
- 5 small cucumbers, chopped
- 3 small avocados, chopped
- ½ teaspoon ground black pepper
- 2 tablespoon olive oil
- 2 tablespoon fresh lemon juice
- ¼ cup fresh cilantro, chopped
- 1 teaspoon sea salt

Directions:

1. Add the cherry tomatoes, cucumbers, avocados, and cilantro into the large mixing bowl and mix well.
2. Mix together olive oil, lemon juice, black pepper, and salt and pour over salad.
3. Mix well and serve immediately.

Nutritional value:
Calories: 442 kcal
Fat: 31 g
Carbs: 30.3 g
Sugar: 4 g
Protein: 2 g
Cholesterol: 0 mg

Healthy Broccoli Salad

Preparation Time: 25 minutes
Cooking Time: 0 minutes
Servings: 6
Ingredients:

- 3 cups broccoli, chopped
- 1 tablespoon apple cider vinegar
- ½ cup greek yogurt
- 2 tablespoon sunflower seeds
- 3 bacon slices, cooked and chopped
- 1/3 cup onion, sliced
- ¼ teaspoon stevia

Directions:

1. In a mixing bowl, mix together the broccoli, onion, and bacon.
2. In a small bowl, mix together the yogurt, vinegar, and stevia and pour over broccoli mixture. Whisk to combine.
3. Sprinkle sunflower seeds on top of the salad.
4. Store salad in the refrigerator for 30 minutes.
5. Serve and enjoy.

Nutritional value:
Calories: 90 kcal
Fat: 9 g
Carbs: 4 g
Sugar: 5 g
Protein: 2 g
Cholesterol: 12 mg

Cauliflower Curry

Preparation Time: 5 minutes
Cooking Time: 5 hours
Servings: 4
Ingredients:

- 1 cauliflower head, florets separated
- 2 carrots, sliced
- 1 red onion, chopped
- ¾ cup coconut milk
- 2 garlic cloves, minced
- 2 tablespoons curry powder
- 1 pinch salt and black pepper
- 1 tablespoon red pepper flakes
- 1 teaspoon garam masala

Directions:

1. In your slow cooker, mix all the ingredients.
2. Cover, cook on high heat for 5 hours, divide into bowls and serve.

Nutritional value:
Calories 160 kcal
Fat 11.5 g
Fiber 5.4 g
Carbs 14.7 g
Protein 3.6 g

Cucumber Bowl with Spices and Greek Yogurt

Preparation Time: 10 minutes
Cooking Time: 20 minutes
Servings: 3
Ingredients:

- 4 cucumbers
- ½ teaspoon chili pepper
- ¼ cup fresh parsley, chopped
- ¾ cup fresh dill, chopped
- 2 tablespoons lemon juice
- ½ teaspoon salt
- ½ teaspoon ground black pepper
- ¼ teaspoon sage
- ½ teaspoon dried oregano
- ⅓ cup Greek yogurt

Directions:

1. Make the cucumber dressing: blend the dill and parsley until you get a green mash.
2. Then combine together the green mash with the lemon juice, salt, ground black pepper, sage, dried oregano, Greek yogurt, and chili pepper.
3. Wisk the mixture well.
4. Chop the cucumbers roughly and combine them with thecucumber dressing. Mix up well.
5. Refrigerate the cucumber for 20 minutes.

Nutritional value:
Calories 114
Fat 1.6
Fiber 4.1
Carbs 23.2
Protein 7.6

Balsamic Caramelized Onions

Preparation Time: 15 minutes
Cooking Time: 30 minutes
Servings: 2
Ingredients:

- 4 medium yellow onions, thinly sliced
- ⅓ cup canola oil
- ¼ cup balsamic vinegar
- 1 tablespoon honey
- ½ teaspoon salt
- Pepper

Directions:

1. Heat oven to 350°F
2. In a non-stick skillet over medium heat sauté thinly cut yellow onions in canola oil for 15 minutes or until they are golden brown.
3. Stir in balsamic vinegar, honey, salt, and pepper. Spread onions in a single layer on a baking sheet and bake for about 15 minutes. Stir and bake for another 15 minutes, or until tender.

Nutritional values:
Calories: 394 kcal
Protein: 0.84 g
Fat: 36.01 g
Carbohydrates: 17.89 g
Calcium, Ca18 mg
Magnesium, Mg11 mg

Lemon Dill Roasted Radishes

Preparation Time: 10 minutes
Cooking Time: 10-15 minutes
Servings: 2
Ingredients:

- 1 bunch radishes halved
- ½ small lemon sliced
- 2 clove garlic roughly minced
- 2 tablespoon butter vegan
- 1 tablespoon olive oil
- 1 teaspoon thyme dried
- 1 pinch salt
- 1 tablespoon dill fresh

Directions:

1. Preheat oven to 400°F
2. Add radishes to a bowl with salt.
3. In a small bowl, whisk together the vegan butter, olive oil, lemon juice, and shallots.
4. Coat radishes generously with butter mixture and place them in a baking dish.
5. Add garlic, thyme, and dill and top with salt and pepper.
6. Roast in the oven for 10-15 minutes.
7. Serve.
8. Store unused portions in the fridge.

Nutritional values:
Calories: 209 kcal
Protein: 1.92 g
Fat: 18.97 gCarbohydrates: 10.68 g
Calcium, Ca107 mg
Magnesium, Mg38 mg

Turmeric Ginger Spiced Cauliflower

Preparation Time: 5 minutes
Cooking Time: 40 minutes
Servings: 4
Ingredients:

- 1 large head of cauliflower, cut into florets
- 1–2 tablespoons olive oil (see notes)
- 1 tablespoon ground turmeric
- 1 teaspoon each: sea salt and chili powder
- ½ teaspoon each: black pepper and ground ginger
- 1 lemon, cut into half slices
- Cilantro, to serve

Directions:

1. Heat the oil in a large saucepan over medium-high heat. Add the cauliflower florets, lemon slices (with the skin), sea salt, and crushed black pepper.
2. Stir well. Add the chili powder, turmeric, ginger, and ground black pepper and stir again. Reduce the heat to medium and cook, stirring frequently, for a further 8–10 minutes. The turmeric will turn the cauliflower golden.
3. When all the water has evaporated, cover the pan with a lid, reduce the heat, and gently cook for another 4–5 minutes, stirring occasionally.
4. Serve immediately with a slice of lemon and a sprig of cilantro.

Nutritional values:
Calories: 61 kcal
Protein: 1.75 g
Fat: 3.77 g
Carbohydrates: 6.58 g
Calcium, Ca23 mg
Magnesium, Mg18 mg

Roasted Garlic Zoodles

Preparation Time: 15 minutes
Cooking Time: 15 minutes
Servings: 4
Ingredients:

- 10 ounces grape tomatoes
- 1 tablespoon grapeseed oil (or any neutral-flavored cooking oil you have on hand)
- 1 teaspoon dried oregano
- Salt to taste
- 2 pounds zucchini, spiralized
- 2 tablespoons fresh lemon juice
- 2 tablespoons extra-virgin olive oil
- 1 teaspoon lemon zest
- 1 large clove garlic, minced
- 3 tablespoons toasted pine nuts

Directions:

1. Preheat oven to 400°F. In a large bowl, toss the tomatoes with the oil, oregano, and a pinch of salt. Transfer to a baking sheet and roast until charred in spots, about 10 minutes.
2. Cook the zoodles in a pot of boiling water until just tender (about 2 minutes) depending on the width of your zoodles.
3. Drain and immediately transfer to a large bowl of ice water to shock them and stop the cooking process. Drain the zoodles again and place them in a large bowl along with the lemon juice (calms the bitter taste from the zucchini), the olive oil, lemon zest, and garlic.
4. Toss to coat. Remove the tomatoes from the oven and let cool slightly (about 5 minutes.) Roughly chop and add them to the bowl along with the pine nuts, sprinkle with salt, and toss again to combine. Serve immediately.

Nutritional values:
Calories: 158 kcal   Protein: 6.8 g Fat: 7.54 g
        Magnesium, Mg82 mg Carbohydrates:
20.93 g
Calcium, Ca61 mg

Heavenly Green Beans and Garlic

Preparation time: 5 minutes
Cooking time: 10 minutes **Servings:** 6-8
Ingredients:

- 2 pounds fresh green beans, trimmed
- 1 tablespoon olive oil
- 3 tablespoons chopped garlic
- ½ teaspoon kosher salt
- ¼ teaspoon ground black pepper

Directions:

1. Heat an indoor or outdoor grill to medium heat.
2. In a small bowl, whisk together the olive oil, garlic, kosher salt, and pepper.
3. Cut the ends off the green beans and reserve for another use or discard.
4. In a large bowl, toss the beans with the olive oil mixture until evenly coated.
5. Lay the beans out on the grill in a single layer.
6. Cover the grill and cook the beans and the garlic for about 5-10 minutes with the lid closed.
7. Toss the beans and continue to cook until they are slightly charred and tender.
8. Move the beans to a serving bowl, drizzle with garlic oil, and season with additional salt if needed.
9. Serve and enjoy.

Nutritional value:
Calories: 128 kcal Protein: 4.5 g Fat: 5.69 g
Carbohydrates: 15.72 g Calcium: 52 mg
Magnesium: 30 mg

Nutty Charred Broccoli

Preparation time: 10 minutes
Cooking time: 15 minutes
Servings: 4
Ingredients

- 4 teaspoons fresh chopped garlic
- 4 teaspoons oil
- 4 cups broccoli florets
- 1 teaspoon Stacey Hawkins' Dash of Desperation Seasoning.

Directions:

1. In a large saucepan, heat the oil and add the garlic. Cook on med-high for 4 minutes, stir often.
2. Add the broccoli and Stacey Hawkins' Dash of Desperation Seasoning, cook on med-high for another 8 minutes, keep stirring.
3. Turn the heat to medium and cook for another 10 minutes till it's nice, brown and tender.
4. Serve hot or cool and store for future use. Enjoy

Nutritional value:
Calories: 51 kcal
Protein: 1.3 g Fat: 4.7 g
Carbohydrates: 1.56 g
Calcium: 43 mg Magnesium: 9 mg

Char-Grilled Cauliflower Steaks

Preparation time: 15 minutes **Cooking time:** 10 minutes **Servings:** 4-6
Ingredients:

- 2 large head cauliflower
- 2 tablespoons olive oil
- 2 lemons, zested and juiced
- 2 cloves garlic, finely minced
- 1 teaspoon honey, use agave syrup to make it vegan
- 2 teaspoons kosher salt
- ¼ teaspoon red pepper flakes
- ¼ cup fresh parsley, chopped
- ¼ cup toasted walnuts, chopped
- Lemon wedges for serving

Directions:

1. Preheat the oven to 400F degrees. You can use larger or smaller heads of cauliflower. For smaller florets, halve the head lengthwise and scoop out the core. For the cauliflower:
2. Preheat the grill or grill pan to medium-high heat. Cut the cauliflower head into 4-6 wedges. Lightly drizzle with olive oil, then season it with half of the kosher salt and pepper flakes. Grill, turning the cauliflower occasionally, until it's tender and golden brown. Cut the cauliflower in half again lengthwise, place it in a mixing bowl. Add the lemon zest, lemon juice, olive oil, parsley, garlic, honey, salt, and pepper to the bowl. Mix everything and let it rest for about 15 minutes to marinate. Bake the cauliflower wedges for about 15-20 minutes at 400F. Watch them to be sure they turn golden brown and crispy.

For the walnuts:

3. Toast the walnuts at 350F for 8-10 minutes. Watch them carefully to avoid burning.
4. Transfer the cauliflower to a platter or serve it right on the baking sheets. Sprinkle the walnuts and add a pinch of kosher salt before serving.

Nutritional value: Calories: 147 kcal Protein: 3.64 g Fat: 11.63 g Carbohydrates: 10.5 g Calcium: 45 mg Magnesium: 32 mg

Roasted Red Radishes a Lean and Green Recipe

Preparation time: 5 minutes
Cooking time: 30 minutes
Servings: 4
Ingredients:

- 4 Cups red and green radish halves, remove stems
- 2 teaspoons cooking oil of your choice
- ½ tablespoon Stacey Hawkins' Dash of Desperation Seasoning

Directions:

1. Preheat oven or toaster oven to 400 to 450 degrees depending on equipment.
2. Take radishes and chop into ¼ square pieces.
3. Spread evenly on top of a baking sheet.
4. Drizzle oil over radishes.
5. Sprinkle Stacey Hawkins' Dash of Desperation Seasoning on top of the radishes.
6. Place on the oven or toaster oven for 30 minutes, stir every ten minutes.
7. Remove from the oven and serve while hot with a piece of toast (to soak up the delicious oil and salt from radishes).
8. Enjoy!

Nutritional value:
Calories: 42 kcal
Protein: 0.84 g
Fat: 2.37 g
Carbohydrates: 4.57 g

Sautéed Summer Vegetables with Lemon and Garlic

Preparation time: 20 minutes
Cooking time: 30 minutes
Servings: 4
Ingredients:

- 1 tablespoon olive oil
- 1 tablespoon butter
- 3 cloves garlic, finely minced
- 1 jalapeno pepper, seeds removed, minced
- 2 medium zucchini, halved lengthwise and sliced
- 1 yellow bell pepper, cut into chunks
- 1 red bell pepper, cut into chunks
- 1 shallot, sliced
- ¼ teaspoon salt
- Freshly ground black pepper to taste
- 1 pinch paprika

Directions:

1. Add the oil and butter to a large frying pan over medium-high heat. Once the butter sizzles add the garlic, jalapeno pepper, and bell peppers, cook for 1 minute.
2. For 18 minutes, stir the vegetables occasionally to keep them from burning until they are softer, lower heat if they begin to burn. In the next 2 minutes, add salt, pepper, and paprika, stir until fragrant.
3. Serve hot or warm.

Nutritional value:
Calories: 310 kcal
Protein: 21.13 g
Fat: 22.7 g
Carbohydrates: 5.07 g
Calcium: 31 mg
Magnesium: 30 mg

Perfect Coleslaw

Preparation time: 30 minutes
Cooking time: 0 minutes
Servings: 4
Ingredients:

- 1 cup mayonnaise
- 4 tablespoons lemon juice
- 3 tablespoons sugar
- Salt and pepper to taste
- 5 cup red and green cabbage, shredded
- 1 cup carrot, shredded
- ¼cup onion, shredded
- ½ cup green bell pepper, sliced (optional)

Directions:

1. Mix the mayonnaise, sugar, lemon juice, salt, and pepper together until it is smooth.
2. Add the cabbage, carrots, red and green bell peppers, and onion.
3. Mix it until all the vegetables are coated with the mayonnaise mixture.
4. Cover it and let it chill for 1 hour before serving.
5. Serve with your favorite lunch.

Nutritional value:

Calories: 282 kcal
Protein: 6 g
Fat: 19.47 g
Carbohydrates: 24.24 g
Calcium: 99 mg
Magnesium: 60 mg

Mashed Garlic Turnips

Preparation Time: 5 minutes
Cooking Time: 10 minutes
Servings: 2
Ingredients:

- 3 cups diced turnip
- 2 cloves garlic, minced
- ¼ cup heavy cream
- 3 tablespoons melted butter
- Salt and pepper to taste

Directions:

1. Boil the turnips until they get tender.
2. Drain and mash the turnips.
3. Add the heavy cream, melted butter, salt, pepper and garlic. Mix well.
4. Serve!

Nutritional value:

Calories: 488 kcal
Carbs: 32 g
Fat: 19 g
Protein: 34 g
Fiber: 20 g

Sophie Haye

Oh so good' Salad

Preparation Time: 5 minutes
Cooking Time: 10 minutes
Servings: 2
Ingredients:

- 6 brussel sprouts
- ½ teaspoon apple cider vinegar
- 1 teaspoon olive or grapeseed oil
- A pinch of salt
- 1 tablespoon freshly grated parmesan

Directions:

1. Slice the clean brussel sprouts in half.
2. Cut thin slices in the opposite direction.
3. Once sliced, cut the roots off and discard.
4. Toss together with the apple cider, oil and salt.
5. Sprinkle the parmesan cheese, combine and enjoy!

Nutritional value:
Calories: 438 kcal
Carbs: 31 g Fat: 23 g
Protein: 24 g
Fiber: 16 g

Green Beans and Garlic

Preparation time: 5 minutes
Cooking time: 5 minutes **Servings:** 4
Ingredients:

- 1 tablespoon olive oil
- 1 ounce green beans, trimmed
- 3 garlic cloves, finely minced
- 1/2 teaspoon sea salt

Directions:

1. In a large pot of salted boiling water, cook the beans until crisp-tender for about 5 minutes. Drain with a colander. Quickly rinse with cold water to stop them from cooking further. Drain well.
2. In a large frying pan over high heat, pour the olive oil and, when it starts to smoke, add the beans and let them sear for 1 minute, stirring constantly.
3. Add the garlic and continue to cook for 1 to 2 more minutes, until the garlic is golden brown and cooked through.
4. Season with salt; then remove from the heat and serve.

Nutritional value:
Calories: 71 kcal   Protein: 0.79 g
Fat: 1.44 g   Carbohydrates: 13.87 g
Calcium: 154 mg   Magnesium: 21 mg

Crispy Zucchini Chips
Preparation Time: 10 minutes
Cooking Time: 4 hours
Servings: 1
Ingredients:
- 1½ cups zucchini
- 1 teaspoon olive oil
- A pinch sea salt

Directions:
1. Heat the oven to 200° F.
2. Prepare two small or one large baking tray using a layer of parchment baking paper. Lightly spray it with cooking oil spray.
3. Slice the zucchini and arrange them in a single layer in the pan.
4. Bake for 3.5 to 4 hours until crispy. Turn the slices for even baking.

Nutritional value:
Calories: 42 kcal
Protein: 0.3 g
Fat: 4.54 g
Carbohydrates: 0.34 g

Thai Roasted Veggies
Preparation Time: 20 minutes
Cooking Time: 6 to 8 hours
Servings: 8
Ingredients:
- 4 large carrots, peeled and cut into chunks
- 2 onions, peeled and sliced
- 6 garlic cloves, peeled and sliced
- 2 parsnips, peeled and sliced
- 2 jalapeño peppers, minced
- ½ cup roasted vegetable broth
- ⅓ cup canned coconut milk
- 3 tablespoons lemon juice
- 2 tablespoons grated fresh ginger root
- 2 teaspoons curry powder

Directions:
1. In a 6-quart slow cooker, mix the carrots, onions, garlic, parsnips, and jalapeño peppers.
2. In a small bowl, mix the vegetable broth, coconut milk, lemonjuice, ginger root, and curry powder until well blended. Pour this mixture into the slow cooker.
3. Cover and cook on low heat for 6 to 8 hours, do it until the vegetables are tender when pierced with a fork.
4. Serve.

Nutritional value:
Calories: 69 kcal
Carbohydrates: 13 g
Sugar: 6 g Fiber: 3 g
Fat: 3g Saturated Fat: 3g
Protein: 1g
Sodium: 95mg

Roasted Squash Puree
Preparation Time: 20 minutes
Cooking Time: 6 to 7 hours
Servings: 8
Ingredients:

- 3 pounds butternut squash, peeled, seeded, and cut into 1-inch pieces
- 1 pound acorn squash, peeled, seeded, and cut into 1-inch pieces
- 2 onions, chopped
- 3 garlic cloves, minced
- 2 tablespoons olive oil
- 1 teaspoon dried marjoram leaves
- ½ teaspoon salt
- ⅛ teaspoon ground black pepper

Directions:

1. In a 6-quart slow cooker, mix all of the ingredients.
2. Cover and cook on low heat for 6 to 7 hours, or until the squash is tender when pierced with a fork.
3. Use a potato masher to mash the squash inside the slow cooker.
4. Serve.

Nutritional value:
Calories: 175 kcal
Carbohydrates: 38 g
Sugar: 1 g
Fiber: 3 g
Fat: 4 g
Saturated Fat: 1 g
Protein: 3 g
Sodium: 149 mg

Three-Bean Medley
Preparation Time: 15 minutes
Cooking Time: 6 to 8 hours **Servings:** 8
Ingredients:

- 1¼ cups dried kidney beans, rinsed and drained
- 1¼ cups dried black beans, rinsed and drained
- 1¼ cups dried black-eyed peas, rinsed and drained
- 1 onion, chopped
- 1 leek, chopped
- 2 garlic cloves, minced
- 2 carrots, peeled and chopped
- 6 cups low-sodium vegetable broth
- 1½ cups water
- ½ teaspoon dried thyme leaves

Directions:

1. In a 6-quart slow cooker, mix all of the ingredients.
2. Put the lid on and cook on low heat for 6 to 8 hours, or until the beans are tender and the liquid is absorbed.
3. Serve.

Nutritional value:
Calories: 284 kcal   Carbohydrates: 56 g Sugar: 6 g Fiber: 19 g Fat: 0 g   Saturated Fat: 0 g Protein: 1 9g   Sodium: 131 mg

Herbed Garlic Black Beans

Preparation Time: 10 minutes
Cooking Time: 7 to 9 hours
Servings: 8
Ingredients:

- 3 cups dried black beans, rinsed and drained
- 2 onions, chopped
- 8 garlic cloves, minced
- 6 cups low-sodium vegetable broth
- ½ teaspoon salt
- 1 teaspoon dried basil leaves
- ½ teaspoon dried thyme leaves
- ½ teaspoon dried oregano leaves

Directions:

1. In a 6-quart slow cooker, mix all the ingredients.
2. Put the lid on and cook on low heat for 7 to 9 hours, or until the beans have absorbed the liquid and are tender.
3. Remove and discard the bay leaf.
4. Serve.

Nutritional value:

Calories: 250 kcal	Carbohydrates: 47 g
Sugar: 3 g	Fiber: 17 g
Fat: 0 g	Saturated Fat: 0 g
Protein: 15 g	Sodium: 253 mg

Roasted Root Vegetables

Preparation Time: 20 minutes
Cooking Time: 6 to 8 hours
Servings: 8
Ingredients:

- 6 carrots, cut into 1-inch chunks
- 2 yellow onions, each cut into 8 wedges
- 2 sweet potatoes, peeled and cut into chunks
- 6 Yukon Gold potatoes, cut into chunks
- 8 whole garlic cloves, peeled
- 4 parsnips, peeled and cut into chunks
- 3 tablespoons olive oil
- 1 teaspoon dried thyme leaves
- ½ teaspoon salt
- ⅛ teaspoon freshly ground black pepper

Directions:

1. In a 6-quart slow cooker, mix all of the ingredients.
2. Put the lid on and cook on low heat for 6 to 8 hours, or until the vegetables are tender.

Nutritional value:

Calories: 214 kcal Carbohydrates: 40 g Sugar: 7 g Fiber: 6 g Fat: 5 g Saturated Fat: 1 g Protein: 4 g Sodium: 201 mg

Crispy-Topped Baked Vegetables

Preparation Time: 10 minutes
Cooking Time: 40 minutes
Servings: 4
Ingredients:

- 2 tablespoon olive oil
- 1 onion, chopped
- 1 celery stalk, chopped
- 2 carrots, grated
- ½ pound turnips, sliced
- 1 cup vegetable broth
- 1 teaspoon turmeric
- Sea salt and black pepper, to taste
- ½ teaspoon liquid smoke
- 1 cup parmesan cheese, shredded
- 2 tablespoon fresh chives, chopped

Directions:

1. Set the oven to 360°F and grease a baking dish with olive oil.
2. Set a skillet over medium heat and add olive oil.
3. Sweat the onion until it gets soft, and place in the turnips, carrots and celery; and cook for 4 minutes.
4. Remove the vegetable mixture to the baking dish.
5. Combine vegetable broth with the turmeric, pepper, liquid smoke, and salt.
6. Spread this mixture over the vegetables.
7. Sprinkle with parmesan cheese and bake for about 30 minutes.
8. Decorate with chives to serve.

Nutritional value:
Calories: 242 kcal
Fats: 16.3 g
Carbohydrates: 8.6 g
Protein: 16.3 g

Greek Salad

Preparation Time: 15 Minutes
Cooking Time: 15 Minutes
Servings: 5
Ingredients:
For Dressing:

- ½ teaspoon black pepper
- ¼ teaspoon salt
- ½ teaspoon oregano
- 1 tablespoon garlic powder
- 2 tablespoons Balsamic
- 1/3 cup olive oil

For Salad:

- ½ cup sliced black olives
- ½ cup chopped parsley, fresh
- 1 small red onion, thin-sliced
- 1 cup cherry tomatoes, sliced
- 1 bell pepper, yellow, chunked
- 1 cucumber, peeled, quarter and slice
- 4 cups chopped romaine lettuce
- ½ teaspoon salt
- 2 tablespoons olive oil

Directions:

1. In a small bowl, blend all of the ingredients for the dressing and let this set in the refrigerator while you make the salad.
2. To assemble the salad, mix together all the ingredients in a large-sized bowl and toss the veggies gently but thoroughly to mix.
3. Serve the salad with the dressing in amounts as desired

Nutrition:
Calories: 234 kcal
Fat: 16.1 g
Protein: 5 g
Carbs: 48 g

Simple Green Beans with Butter

Preparation Time: 2 minutes
Cooking Time: 10 minutes
Servings: 4
Ingredients:

- ¾ pound green beans, cleaned
- 1 tablespoon balsamic vinegar
- ¼ teaspoon kosher salt
- ½ teaspoon mixed peppercorns, freshly cracked
- 1 tablespoon butter
- 2 tablespoons toasted sesame seeds, to serve

Directions:

1. Set your Air Fryer to cook at 390°F.
2. Mix the green beans with all of the ingredients, apart from the sesame seeds and put them into the Air Fryer. Set the timer for 10 minutes.
3. Meanwhile, toast the sesame seeds in a small-sized nonstick skillet; make sure to stir continuously.
4. Serve sautéed green beans on a nice serving platter sprinkled with toasted sesame seeds. Bon appétit!

Nutritional value:

Calories: 73 kcal   Fat: 3.0g
Carbs: 6.1g
Protein: 1.6g
Sugars: 1.2g   Fiber: 2.1g

Creamy Cauliflower and Broccoli

Preparation Time: 4 minutes
Cooking Time: 16 minutes
Servings: 6
Ingredients:

- 1 pound cauliflower florets
- 1 pound broccoli florets
- 2 ½ tablespoons sesame oil
- ½ teaspoon smoked cayenne pepper
- ¾ teaspoon sea salt flakes
- 1 tablespoon lemon zest, grated
- ½ cup Colby cheese, shredded

Directions:

1. Prepare the cauliflower and broccoli using your favorite steaming method. Then, drain them well; add the sesame oil, cayenne pepper, and salt flakes.
2. Air-fry at 390° F for approximately 16 minutes—make sure to check the vegetables halfway through the cooking time.
3. Afterwards, stir in the lemon zest and Colby cheese; toss to coat well and serve immediately!

Nutritional value:

Calories: 133 kcal
Fat: 9.0g
Carbs: 9.5g
Protein: 5.9g
Sugars: 3.2g
Fiber: 3.6g

Spicy Zesty Broccoli with Tomato Sauce

Preparation Time: 5 minutes
Cooking Time: 15 minutes
Servings: 6
Ingredients:
For the Broccoli Bites:

- 1 medium-sized head broccoli, broken into florets
- ½ teaspoon lemon zest, freshly grated
- ⅓ teaspoon fine sea salt
- ½ teaspoon hot paprika
- 1 teaspoon shallot powder
- 1 teaspoon porcini powder
- ½ teaspoon granulated garlic
- ⅓ teaspoon celery seeds
- 1 ½ tablespoons olive oil

For the Hot Sauce:

1. ½ cup tomato sauce
2. 1 tablespoon balsamic vinegar
3. ½ teaspoon ground allspice

Directions:

1. Toss all the ingredients for the broccoli bites in a mixing bowl, covering the broccoli florets on all sides.
2. Cook them in the preheated Air Fryer at 360°F for 13–15 minutes. In the meantime, mix all ingredients for the hot sauce.
3. Pause your Air Fryer, mix the broccoli with the prepared sauce and cook for a further 3 minutes. Bon appétit!

Nutritional value:
Calories: 70 kcal
Fat: 3.8g
Carbs: 5.8g
Protein: 2g
Sugars: 6.6g
Fiber: 1.5g

Cheese Stuffed Mushrooms with Horseradish Sauce

Preparation Time: 3 minutes
Cooking Time: 12 minutes
Servings: 5
Ingredients:

- ½ cup parmesan cheese, grated
- 2 cloves garlic, pressed
- 2 tablespoons fresh coriander, chopped
- ⅓ teaspoon kosher salt
- ½ teaspoon crushed red pepper flakes
- 1 ½ tablespoons olive oil
- 20 medium-sized mushrooms (cut off the stems)
- ½ cup Gorgonzola cheese, grated
- ¼ cup low-fat mayonnaise
- 1 teaspoon prepared horseradish, well-drained
- 1 tablespoon fresh parsley, finely chopped

Directions:

1. Mix the parmesan cheese together with the garlic, coriander, salt, red pepper, and the olive oil; mix to combine well.
2. Stuff the mushroom caps with the cheese filling. Top with grated Gorgonzola.
3. Place the mushrooms in the Air Fryer grill pan and slide them into the machine. Grill them at 380°F for 8–12 minutes or until the stuffing is warmed through.
4. Meanwhile, prepare the horseradish sauce by mixing the mayonnaise, horseradish and parsley. Serve the horseradish sauce with the warm fried mushrooms. Enjoy!

Nutritional value:
Calories: 180 kcal
Fat: 13.2g
Carbs: 6.2g
Protein: 8.6g
Sugars: 2.1g
Fiber: 1g

Broccoli with Herbs and Cheese
Preparation Time: 8 minutes
Cooking Time: 17 minutes
Servings: 4
Ingredients:

- ⅓ cup grated yellow cheese
- 1 large-sized head broccoli, stemmed and cut into small florets
- 2 ½ tablespoons canola oil
- 2 teaspoons dried rosemary
- 2 teaspoons dried basil
- Salt and ground black pepper, to taste

Directions:

1. Bring a medium pan filled with a lightly salted water to a boil. Then, boil the broccoli florets for about 3 minutes.
2. Drain the broccoli florets well; toss them with the canola oil, rosemary, basil, salt and black pepper.
3. Set the oven to 390°F; arrange the seasoned broccoli in the cooking basket; set the timer for 17 minutes. Toss the broccoli halfway through the cooking process.
4. Serve warm topped with grated cheese and enjoy!

Nutritional value:
Calories: 111 kcal
Fat: 2.1g
Carbs: 3.9g
Protein: 8.9g
Sugars: 1.2g
Fiber: 0.4g

Family Favorite Stuffed Mushrooms
Preparation Time: 4 minutes
Cooking Time: 12 minutes
Servings: 2
Ingredients:

- 2 teaspoons cumin powder
- 4 garlic cloves, peeled and minced
- 1 small onion, peeled and chopped
- 18 medium-sized white mushrooms
- Fine sea salt and freshly ground black pepper, to taste
- A pinch ground allspice
- 2 tablespoons olive oil

Directions:

1. First, clean the mushrooms; remove the middle stalks from the mushrooms to prepare the "shells".
2. Grab a mixing dish and thoroughly combine the remaining items. Fill the mushrooms with the prepared mixture.
3. Cook the mushrooms at 345°F and heat for 12 minutes. Enjoy!

Nutritional value:
Calories: 179 kcal   Fat: 14.7g
Carbs: 8.5g
Protein: 5.5g
Sugars: 4.6g
Fiber: 2.6g

Grilled Eggplants

Preparation Time: 10 minutes
Cooking Time: 10 minutes
Servings: 4
Ingredients:

- 1 large eggplant, cut into thick slices
- Salt and pepper to taste
- 1 teaspoon smoked paprika
- 1 tablespoon coconut flour
- 1 teaspoon lime juice
- 1 tablespoon olive oil

Directions:

1. Coat the eggplants in smoked paprika, salt, pepper, lime juice, coconut flour, and let it sit for 10 minutes.
2. Add the olive oil on a grilling pan
3. Grill the eggplants for 3 minutes on each side.
4. Serve.

Nutritional value:

Fat: 0.1 g
Sodium: 1.6 mg
Carbohydrates: 4.8 g
Fiber: 2.4 g
Sugars: 2.9 g
Protein: 0.8 g

Sweet Potato Casserole

Preparation Time: 20 minutes
Cooking Time: 1 hour
Servings: 8
Ingredients:

- Potatoes (3 lbs., sweet, peeled, chopped)
- Greek yogurt (1 cup, nonfat)
- Cinnamon (1/2 tbsp, ground)
- Nutmeg (1/8 tsp., ground)
- Sea salt (1/4 tsp.)
- Egg whites (6 tbsp)
- Butter (1 tbsp, melted)
- Pecans (1/2 cup, chopped)
- Marshmallows (1/2 cup, miniature)
- Sugar (dash, light brown, for sprinkling)

Directions:

1. Heat your oven to 375 degrees Fahrenheit.
2. Place the potatoes (sweet) into a saucepan (large) over medium high heat.
3. Cover potatoes using water then bring to a boil, boil for approximately 30 minutes until soft.
4. Drain potatoes then place potatoes back into the saucepan.
5. Add the Greek yogurt, cinnamon (ground), nutmeg (base) and sea salt (dash) into the potatoes.
6. Stir well until coated (evenly).
7. Add in the butter (melted) and egg whites then bring to a stir once more.
8. Transfer potato mixture into a casserole dish (large).
9. Place into oven then bake for approximately 30 minutes. Remove from heat then top with the pecans (chopped) and miniature marshmallows.
10. Place back into oven to bake for an additional 10 minutes until marshmallows are browned.

Nutritional value:

Calories: 266 kcal
Protein: 2.9 g
Carbohydrates: 30.1 g
Dietary Fiber: 1.9 g

Baked Cheesy Eggplant

Preparation Time: 20 minutes
Cooking Time: 1 hour and 15 minutes
Servings: 6
Ingredients:

- Eggplant (1, fresh)
- Tomato (1, 16 can, chopped)
- Tomato sauce (2, 8 oz. can)
- Cheddar cheese (6 oz., shredded)
- Onion (1, chopped)
- Oregano (dash, dried)
- Salt (2 tsp.)
- Italian seasoning (dash)
- Basil (dried, for taste)
- Thyme (dried, for flavor)
- Garlic (2-3 tsp., powdered)
- Black pepper (1/2 tsp.)

Directions:

1. Slice eggplant (fresh) into thin slices then season using a dash of salt.
2. Next, set aside in a colander for roughly 30 minutes then pat dry using a few paper towels.
3. Rinse under warm running water and thoroughly slice eggplant into quarters.
4. Place a layer of the eggplant (quartered) into a baking dish (large).
5. Cover layer using the tomatoes (chopped) and tomato sauce (1 can).
6. Add 1/2 of the cheese over the top and repeat layers with the remaining cheese (shredded) over the top.
7. Place eggplant into the oven to bake for approximately 45 minutes at 350 degrees Fahrenheit until eggplant is soft.

Nutritional value:
Calories: 120 kcal
Protein: 11.7 g
Carbohydrates: 15.4 g
Dietary Fiber: 5.4 g

Light Paprika Moussaka

Preparation Time: 15 minutes
Cooking Time: 45 minutes
Servings: 3
Ingredients:

- 1 eggplant, trimmed
- 1 cup ground chicken
- ⅓ cup white onion, diced
- 3 ounce Cheddar cheese, shredded
- 1 potato, sliced
- 1 teaspoon olive oil
- 1 teaspoon salt
- ½ cup milk
- 1 tablespoon butter
- 1 tablespoon ground paprika
- 1 tablespoon Italian seasoning
- 1 teaspoon tomato paste

Directions:

1. Slice the eggplant lengthwise and sprinkle it with salt.
2. Pour the olive oil in the skillet and add sliced potato.
3. Roast the potato for 2 minutes from each side.
4. Then transfer it to the plate.
5. Put the eggplant in the skillet and roast it for 2 minutes from each side too.
6. Pour the milk in the pan and bring it to boil.
7. Add the tomato paste, Italian seasoning, paprika, butter, and the Cheddar cheese.
8. Then mix up together the onion with the ground chicken.
9. Arrange the sliced potato in the casserole in one layer.
10. Then add ½ part of all sliced eggplants.
11. Spread the eggplants with ½ part of chicken mixture.
12. Then add remaining eggplants.
13. Pour the milk mixture over the eggplants.
14. Bake moussaka for 30 minutes at 355°F.

Nutritional value:
Calories 387 kcal
Fat 21.2 g
Fiber 8.9 g Carbs 26.3 g
Protein 25.4 g

Chapter 10:

Other Lean and Green Delicious recipes

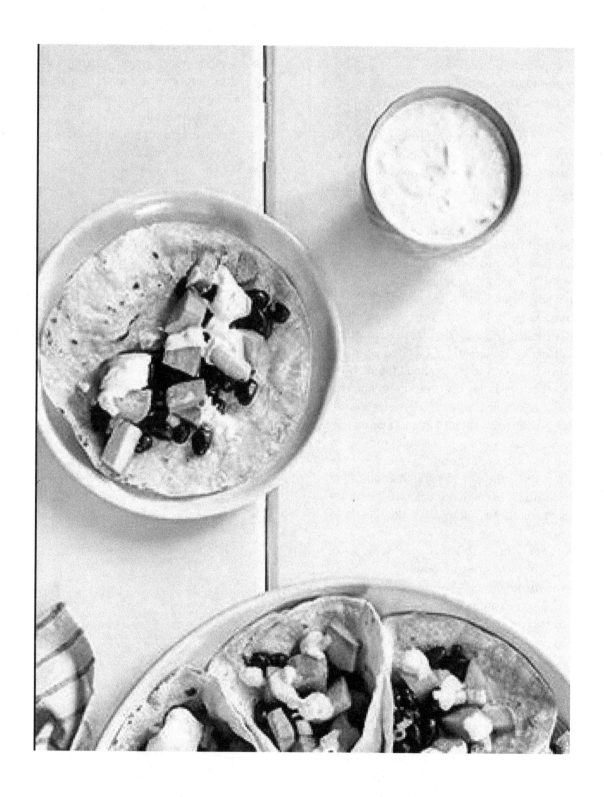

Tofu Power Bowl

Preparation Time: 5 minutes
Cooking Time: 25 minutes
Servings: 8
Ingredients:

- 15 ounces extra-firm tofu
- 2 teaspoon rice vinegar
- 2 tablespoons soy sauce
- 1 teaspoon sesame oil
- ½ cup grated cauliflower
- ½ cup grated eggplant
- ½ cup chopped kale

Directions:

1. Place the tofu strips in multiple layers of paper towel on top of a cutting board. Place another clean paper towel on top of the tofu. Place a weight on top of this second layer (this can be a large plate with canned foods on top or hardcover books). Let it sit for at least 15 minutes, and then cut the tofu into 1-inch cubes.
2. Combine both the vinegar and soy sauce in a small bowl and whisk together
3. Get a large skillet and heat the sesame oil in it. Place the cubed tofu to cover one half of the skillet, and the cubed eggplant should cover the other half. Cook both together until they become slightly brown and tender in about 10-12 minutes. Remove it from the skillet and keep aside. Now, add kale and sauté until they become wilted in about 3-5 minutes.
4. Microwave the already grated cauliflower in a small bowl with one teaspoon of water for about 3-4 minutes till it becomes tender.
5. Arrange the cauliflower rice with tofu, eggplant, and kale in a bowl.

Nutritional value:
Calories: 320 kcal Protein: 43g
Carbohydrate: 13 g Fat: 11 g

Delicious Zucchini Quiche

Preparation Time: 25 minutes
Cooking Time: 1 hour
Servings: 8
Ingredients:

- 6 eggs
- 2 medium zucchini, shredded
- ½ teaspoon dried basil
- 2 garlic cloves, minced
- 1 tablespoon dry onion, minced
- 2 tablespoon parmesan cheese, grated
- 2 tablespoon fresh parsley, chopped
- ½ cup olive oil
- 1 cup cheddar cheese, shredded
- ¼ cup coconut flour
- ¾ cup almond flour
- ½ teaspoon salt

Directions:

1. Preheat the oven to 350°F. Grease a 9-inch pie pan and set aside.
2. Squeeze excess liquid from zucchini.
3. Add all ingredients to a large bowl and mix until well combined. Pour it into the prepared cake pan.
4. Bake in a preheated oven for 45-60 minutes or until cooked through.
5. Remove from the oven and let it cool completely.
6. Slice and serve.

Nutritional value:
Calories: 288 kcal Fat: 23 g Carbs: 5 g Sugar: 6 g
Protein: 11 g Cholesterol: 139 mg

Asparagus and Crabmeat Frittata

Preparation Time: 10 minutes
Cooking Time: 30 minutes
Servings: 4
Ingredients:

- 21/2 tbsp. extra virgin olive oil
- 2 pound asparagus
- 1 teaspoon salt
- 1 1/2 tsp. black pepper
- 2 teaspoon sweet paprika
- 1 pound. lump crabmeat
- 1 tablespoon finely cut chives
- 1/4 cup basil chopped
- 4 cups liquid egg substitute

Directions:

8. Remove the tough ends of the asparagus and cut it into bite-sized pieces.
9. Preheat an oven to 375°F. In a 12-Inch to a 14-inch ovenproof, non-stick skillet, warm the olive oil and sweat the asparagus until tender.
10. Season with pepper, paprika, and salt. In a mixing bowl, add the chives, crab and basil meat.
11. Pour in the liquid egg substitute and mix until combined.
12. Pour the crab, egg mixture into the skillet with the cooked asparagus, and stir to combine.
13. Bake over low to medium heat until the eggs start bubbling.
14. Place the skillet in the oven and bake for about 15-20 minutes until the eggs are golden brown.
15. Serve the dish warm.

Nutritional value:
Calories: 340 kcal Protein: 50 g
Carbohydrates: 14 g
Fats: 10 g

Ancho Tilapia on Cauliflower Rice

Preparation Time: 15 minutes
Cooking Time: 30 minutes
Servings: 4
Ingredients:

- 2 pounds. tilapia
- 1 teaspoon lime juice
- 1 teaspoon salt
- 1 tablespoons ground ancho pepper
- 1 teaspoon ground cumin
- 1 ½ tablespoons extra virgin olive oil
- ¼ up toasted pumpkin seeds
- 6 cups cauliflower rice minutes
- 1 cup coarsely chopped fresh cilantro

Directions:

1. Preheat oven to 450°F. Dress tilapia with limejuice and set aside.
2. Combine cumin, ancho pepper, and salt in a bowl.
3. Season tilapia with spice mixture.
4. Lay tilapia on a baking sheet or casserole dish and bake for 7 minutes.
5. In the meantime, in a big skillet, sweat the cauliflower rice in olive oil until tender, about 2-3 minutes.
6. Blend the pumpkin seeds and cilantro into the rice.
7. Dismiss from heat, and serve

Nutritional value:
Calories: 350 Cal
Fats: 13 g
Carbohydrates: 10 g
Protein: 51 g

Rosemary Cauliflower Rolls
Preparation Time: 10 minutes
Cooking Time: 30 minutes **Servings:** 3
Ingredients:
- 1/3 cup almond flour
- 4 cups riced cauliflower
- 1/3 cup reduced-fat, shredded mozzarella or cheddar cheese
- 2 eggs
- 2 tablespoon fresh rosemary, finely chopped - ½ teaspoon salt

Directions:
1. Preheat the oven to 400°F
2. Combine all the listed ingredients in a medium-sized bowl
3. Scoop cauliflower mixture into 12 evenly-sized rolls/biscuits onto a lightly-greased and foil-lined baking sheet.
4. Bake until it turns golden brown, which should be achieved in about 30 minutes.

Note: if you want to have the outside of the rolls/biscuits crisp, then broil for some minutes before serving.

Nutritional value:
Calories: 254 kcal
Protein: 24 g
Carbohydrate: 7 g
Fat: 8 g

Greek Style Quesadillas
Preparation Time: 10 minutes
Cooking Time: 10 minutes
Servings: 4
Ingredients:
- 4 whole wheat tortillas
- 1 cup Mozzarella cheese, shredded
- 1 cup fresh spinach, chopped
- 2 tablespoon Greek yogurt
- 1 egg, beaten
- ¼ cup green olives, sliced
- 1 tablespoon olive oil
- 1/3 cup fresh cilantro, chopped

Directions:
1. In a bowl, combine together the Mozzarella cheese, spinach, yogurt, egg, olives, and cilantro.
2. Then pour olive oil in the skillet.
3. Place one tortilla in the skillet and spread it with Mozzarella mixture.
4. Top it with the second tortilla and spread it with cheese mixture again.
5. Then place the third tortilla and spread it with all remaining cheese mixture.
6. Cover it with the last tortilla and fry it for 5 minutes each side over medium heat.

Nutritional value:
Calories 193 kcal
Fat 7.7 g Fiber 3.2 g
Carbs 23.6 g
Protein 8.3 g

Stuffed Bell Peppers with Quinoa
Preparation Time: 10 minutes
Cooking Time: 35 minutes
Servings: 2
Ingredients:

- 2 bell peppers
- ⅓ cup quinoa
- 3 ounces chicken stock
- ¼ cup onion, diced
- ½ teaspoon salt
- ¼ teaspoon tomato paste
- ½ teaspoon dried oregano
- ⅓ cup sour cream
- 1 teaspoon paprika

Directions:

1. Trim the bell peppers and remove the seeds.
2. Then combine together the chicken stock and quinoa in the pan.
3. Add salt and boil the ingredients for 10 minutes or until quinoa absorb all the liquid.
4. Then combine together the cooked quinoa with dried oregano, tomato paste, and onion.
5. Fill the bell peppers with the quinoa mixture and arrange in the casserole mold.
6. Add sour cream and bake the peppers for 25 minutes at 365°F.
7. Serve the cooked peppers with sour cream sauce from the casserole mold.

Nutritional value:
Calories 237 kcal
Fat 10.3 g Fiber 4.5 g
Carbs 31.3 g
Protein 6.9 g

Mediterranean Burrito
Preparation Time: 10 minutes
Cooking Time: 0 minutes
Servings: 2
Ingredients:

- 2 wheat tortillas
- 2 ounces red kidney beans, canned, drained
- 2 tablespoons hummus
- 2 teaspoons tahini sauce
- 1 cucumber
- 2 lettuce leaves
- 1 tablespoon lime juiced
- 1 teaspoon olive oil
- ½ teaspoon dried oregano

Directions:

1. Mash the red kidney beans until you get a puree.
2. Then spread the wheat tortillas with beans mash from one side.
3. Add hummus and tahini sauce.
4. Cut the cucumber into the wedges and place them over tahini sauce.
5. Then add lettuce leaves.
6. Make the dressing: mix up together olive oil, dried oregano, and lime juice.
7. Drizzle the lettuce leaves with the dressing and wrap the wheat tortillas in the shape of burritos.

Nutritional value:
Calories 288 kcal
Fat 10.2 g
Fiber 14.6 g
Carbs 38.2 g
Protein 12.5 g

Cloud Bread

Preparation Time: 25 minutes
Cooking Time: 35 minutes
Servings: 3
Ingredients:

- ½ cup Fat-free 0% Plain Greek Yogurt
- 3 Eggs, Separated
- 16 teaspoon Cream of Tartar
- 1 Packet sweetener (a granulated sweetener just like stevia)

Directions:

1. For about 30 minutes before making this meal, place the Kitchen Aid Bowl and the whisk attachment in the freezer.
2. Preheat the oven to 300°F
3. Remove the mixing bowl and whisk attachment from the freezer
4. Separate the eggs. Now put the egg whites in the Kitchen Aid Bowl, and they should be in a different medium-sized bowl.
5. In the medium-sized bowl containing the yolks, mix in the sweetener and yogurt.
6. In the bowl containing the egg white, add in the cream of tartar. Beat this mixture until the egg whites turn to stiff peaks.
7. Now, take the egg yolk mixture and carefully fold it into the egg whites. Be cautious and avoid over-stirring.
8. Place baking paper on a baking tray and spray with cooking spray.
9. Scoop out 6 equally-sized "blobs" of the "dough" onto the parchment paper.
10. Bake for about 25–35 minutes (make sure you check when it is 25 minutes, in some ovens, they are done at this timestamp). You will know they are done as they will get brownish at the top and have some crack.
11. Most people like them cold against being warm
12. Most people like to re-heat in a toast oven or toaster to get them a little bit crispy.
13. Your serving size should be about 2 pieces.

Nutritional value:
Calories: 234 kcal   Protein: 23g Carbs: 5g
Fiber: 8g   Sodium: 223g

Broccoli Cheddar Breakfast Bake

Preparation Time: 10 minutes
Cooking Time: 45 minutes
Servings: 4
Ingredients:

- 9 eggs
- 6 cups small broccoli florets
- ¼ teaspoon salt
- 1 cup unsweetened almond milk
- ¼ teaspoon cayenne pepper
- ¼ teaspoon ground pepper
- Cooking spray
- 4 ounces shredded, reduced-fat cheddar

Directions:

1. Preheat the oven to about 375°F
2. In your large microwave-safe, add broccoli and 2 to 3 tablespoon of water. Microwave on high heat for 4 minutes or until it becomes tender. Now transfer the broccoli to a colander to drain excess liquid
3. Get a medium-sized bowl and whisk the milk, eggs, and seasonings together.
4. Set the broccoli neatly on the bottom of a lightly greased 13 x 9-inch baking dish. Sprinkle the cheese gently on the broccoli and pour the egg mixture on top of it.
5. Bake for about 45 minutes or until the center is set and the top forms a light brown crust.

Nutritional value:
Calories: 290 kcal
Protein: 25g
Carbohydrate: 8g
Fat: 18 g

Cheese-Stuffed Jalapeño Peppers

Preparation Time: 10 minutes
Cooking Time: 10 minutes
Servings: 1
Ingredients:

- 3–4 geeen Jalapeños
- ¼ cup 2% reduced-fat Mexican Three Cheese Blend
- 2 Light laughing cow cream cheese
- Optional: ⅛ teaspoon Worcestershire sauce
- 2 tbsp Grated-reduced-fat parmesan cheese

Directions:

1. Preheat the oven at 400° Fahrenheit.
2. Prepare the jalapenos by slicing them into halves—lengthwise. Discard the insides (membranes and seeds). Boil them in a large saucepan of water for five to ten minutes. They will become milder - the longer you cook. Drain and rinse in cold water.
3. Combine the cheddar cheese, Worcestershire sauce, and cream cheese. Scoop two teaspoonfuls into each piece of jalapeño with a dusting of the parmesan cheese.
4. Arrange them onto a greased baking tray. Bake them until the cheese is melted (5-10 min.). Serve warm.

Nutritional value:
Calories: 4390 kcal
Protein: 127.32 g
Fat: 329.99 g
Carbohydrates: 243.1 g

Lasagna Spaghetti Squash

Preparation Time: 30 minutes
Cooking Time: 90 minutes
Servings: 6
Ingredients:

- 25 slices mozzarella cheese
- 40 ounces Rao's Marinara sauce
- 30 ounces whole-milk ricotta cheese
- 44 ounces spaghetti squash, cooked
- 4 pounds ground beef

Directions:

1. Preheat your fryer to 375°F.
2. Slice the spaghetti squash and place it face down inside a fryer pan. Fill it with water until covered.
3. Bake for 45 minutes until the skin is soft.
4. Cook the meat until browned.
5. In a large frying pan, heat the browned meat and marinara sauce. Set aside when it gets warm.
6. Scrape the flesh off the cooked squash to resemble strands of spaghetti.
7. Layer the lasagna in a large greased pan, alternating between layers of spaghetti squash, meat sauce, mozzarella, ricotta. Repeat until everything has been used.
8. Bake for 30 minutes and serve!

Nutritional value:
Calories: 508 kcal
Carbs: 32 g
Fat: 8 g
Protein: 22 g
Fiber: 21 g

Sophie Haye

Roasted Cauliflower Hummus
Preparation time: 5 minutes
Cooking time: 35 minutes **Servings:** 12
Ingredients:
- 4 cups cauliflower florets
- ¼ cup extra virgin olive oil
- ½ cup tahini
- 2 cloves garlic, minced or chopped
- 2 tablespoons lemon juice
- 1 teaspoon sea salt
- 1 ½ teaspoon cumin
- ¼ teaspoon paprika
- 3-5 tablespoon Water

Directions:
1. Roast a whole cauliflower (leave the skin on) in the oven for 30-35 minutes or until soft and brown. Let it cool.
2. Remove the cauliflower from the head and put it in the food processor with the rest of the ingredients. Process it until smooth.
3. Add more water if necessary, to achieve the desired consistency and taste. Garnish with chopped parsley and olives.
4. Serve.

Nutritional value:
Calories: 212 kcal
Protein: 6 g
Fat: 17.96 g
Carbohydrates: 10.51 g
Calcium: 131 mg
Magnesium: 39 mg

Fragrant Cauliflower Rice
Preparation time: 10 minutes
Cooking time: 15 minutes
Servings: 6
Ingredients:
- ⅓ cup ghee
- 2 garlic cloves, finely chopped
- ½-inch ginger, finely chopped
- 1 teaspoon coriander seeds
- ½ teaspoon cumin seeds
- ½ teaspoon brown mustard seeds
- ½ teaspoon yellow mustard seeds
- ½ teaspoon turmeric ground
- 26 ounces cauliflower processed into rice
- 1 or 2 teaspoons salt
- ½ teaspoon Pepper
- 2 tablespoons cilantro, chopped

Directions:
1. Melt the ghee in a pan over medium heat, add the garlic, then the ginger, and sauté until the raw smell disappears.
2. Stir in the coriander seeds, cumin seeds, and mustard seeds, and sauté for 1 minute.
3. Stir in the turmeric, cauliflower rice, salt, and pepper. Cover and cook for 10 minutes.
4. Uncover it and mix it gently. Cook for another 5 minutes with the lid on. Then uncover it and toss the cilantro.
5. Serve hot.
6. Serve with yogurt, raita, Iftar meal, or any kind of meal as desired.

Nutritional value: Calories: 71 kcal Protein: 0.79 g Fat: 1.44 gCarbohydrates: 13.87 g alcium: 154 mg Magnesium: 21 mg

Cauliflower Crust Pizza

Preparation Time: 20 minutes
Cooking Time: 45 minutes **Servings:** 4
Ingredients:

- 1 cauliflower (cut into smaller portions)
- ¼ grated parmesan cheese
- 1 egg
- 1 teaspoon italian seasoning
- ¼ teaspoon kosher salt
- 2 cups freshly grated mozzarella
- ¼ cup spicy pizza sauce
- Basil leaves, for decorating

Directions:

1. Begin by preheating the oven while using the parchment paper to rim the baking sheet.
2. Process the cauliflower into a fine powder, and then transfer to a bowl, before putting it into the microwave.
3. Leave for about 5-6 minutes till it gets soft.
4. Transfer the microwave cauliflower to a clean and dry kitchen towel.
5. Leave it to cool off.
6. When cold, use the kitchen towel to wrap the cauliflower and then get rid of all the moisture by wringing the towel. Continue squeezing until water is gone completely.
7. Put the cauliflower, italian seasoning, parmesan cheese, egg, salt, and 1 cup of mozzarella. Stir very well until well combined.
8. Transfer the combined mixture to the baking sheet previously prepared, pressing it into a 10-inch round shape.
9. Bake for 10-15 minutes until it becomes golden.
10. Take the baked crust out of the oven and use the spicy pizza sauce and mozzarella (the leftover 1 cup) to top it.
11. Bake again for 10 more minutes until the cheese melts and looks bubbly.
12. Decorate using fresh basil leaves.

Note: you can also enjoy this with salad.

Nutritional value: Calories: 74 kcal
Carbohydrates: 4 g Protein: 6 g   Fat: 4 g
Fiber: 2 g

Maple Lemon Tempeh Cubes

Preparation Time: 10 minutes
Cooking Time: 30 to 40 minutes
Servings: 4
Ingredients:

- 1 packet tempeh
- 2 to 3 teaspoons coconut oil
- 3 tablespoons lemon juice
- 2 teaspoons maple syrup
- 1 to 2 teaspoons Bragg's Liquid Aminos or low-sodium tamari (optional)
- 2 teaspoons water
- ¼ teaspoon dried basil
- ¼ teaspoon powdered garlic
- Black pepper to taste

Directions:

1. Heat the oven to 400 ° C.
2. Cut your tempeh block into small squares.
3. Heat coconut oil over medium to high heat in a non-stick skillet.
4. When melted and heated, add the tempeh and cook on one side for 2-4 minutes, or until the tempeh turns down into a golden-brown color.
5. Flip the tempeh bits, and cook for another 2-4 minutes.
6. Mix the lemon juice, tamari, maple syrup, basil, water, garlic, and black pepper while the tempeh is cooking.
7. Drizzle the mixture over the tempeh, then swirl to cover it all.
8. Sauté for 2-3 minutes, then turn the tempeh and sauté 1-2 minutes more.
9. The tempeh should be soft and orange on both sides.

Nutritional value:
Carbohydrates: 22 Cal   Fiber: 9 g
Fats: 17 g
Sugar: 5 g
Protein: 21 g

Bok Choy with Tofu Stir Fry
Preparation Time: 15 minutes
Cooking Time: 15 minutes
Servings: 4
Ingredients:
- 1 pound super-firm tofu, drained and pressed
- 1 tablespoon coconut oil
- 1 garlic clove, minced
- 3 heads baby bok choy, chopped
- Low-sodium vegetable broth
- 2 teaspoons maple syrup
- Bragg's liquid aminos
- 1 to 2 teaspoons sambal oelek (similar to chili sauce)
- 1 Scallion or green onion, chopped
- 1 teaspoon freshly grated ginger
- Quinoa or rice for serving

Directions:
1. With paper towels, press the tofu dry and cut it into tiny pieces of about ½ inch wide.
2. Heat coconut oil in a wide skillet till it gets warm.
3. Remove tofu and stir-fry until painted softly.
4. Stir-fry for 1-2 minutes before the choy of the bok starts to wilt.
5. When this happens apply the vegetable broth and all the remaining ingredients to the skillet.
6. Hold the mixture stir-frying until all components are well coated, and the bulk of the liquid evaporates, around 5-6 minutes.
7. Serve over brown rice or quinoa.

Nutritional value:
Calories: 263.7 kcal Fat 4.2 g
Cholesterol: 0.3 mg Sodium: 683.6 mg
Potassium: 313.7 mg Carbohydrate: 35.7 g

Quinoa With Vegetables
Preparation Time: 10 minutes
Cooking Time: 5 to 6 hours **Servings:** 8
Ingredients:
- 2 cups quinoa, rinsed and drained
- 2 onions, chopped
- 2 carrots, peeled and sliced
- 1 cup sliced cremini mushrooms
- 3 garlic cloves, minced
- 4 cups low-sodium vegetable broth
- ½ teaspoon salt
- 1 teaspoon dried marjoram leaves
- ⅛ teaspoon freshly ground black pepper

Directions:
1. In a 6-quart slow cooker, mix all of the ingredients.
2. Put the lid on and cook on low heat for 5 to 6 hours, or until the quinoa and vegetables are tender.
3. Stir the mixture and serve.

Nutritional value:
Calories: 204kcal
Carbohydrates: 35 g
Sugar: 4 g
Fiber: 4 g
Fat: 3 g
Saturated Fat: 0 g
Protein: 7 g
Sodium: 229 mg

Creamy Spinach and Mushroom Lasagna

Preparation Time: 60 minutes
Cooking Time: 20 minutes
Servings: 6
Ingredients:

- 10 lasagna noodles
- 1 package whole milk ricotta
- 2 packages of frozen chopped spinach
- 4 cups mozzarella cheese, divided and shredded
- ¾ cup grated fresh Parmesan
- 3 tablespoons chopped fresh parsley leaves (optional)
  For the Sauce:
- 1/4 cup butter, unsalted
- 2 garlic cloves
- 1 pound of thinly sliced cremini mushroom
- 1 diced onion
- ¼ cup flour
- 4 cups milk, kept at room temperature
- 1 teaspoon basil, dried
- Pinch of nutmeg
- Salt and freshly ground black pepper, to taste

Directions:

1. Preheat the oven to 352°F.
2. To make the sauce, on medium heat, melt the butter and add the garlic, mushrooms and onion. Cook and stir occasionally until it becomes tender, for about 3-4 minutes.
3. Add in the flour until lightly browned, it takes about 1 minute for it to become brown.
4. Next, add in the milk gradually, and cook, always whisking, for about 2-3 minute till it becomes thickened. Add in the basil, oregano and nutmeg, season with salt and pepper for taste;
5. Then set aside.
6. In another pot of boiling salted water, cook the lasagna noodles according to the package instructions.
7. Spread 1 cup mushroom sauce onto the bottom of a baking dish, top it with 4

lasagna noodles, ½ of the spinach, 1 cup mozzarella cheese and ¼ cup Parmesan.
8. Repeat this process with the remaining noodles, mushroom sauce and cheeses.
9. Place it into the oven and bake for 35-45 minutes, or until it starts bubbling. Then boil for 2-3 minutes until it becomes brown and translucent.
10. Let it cool for 15 minutes.
11. Serve it with garnished parsley (optional)

Nutritional value:
Calories: 488.3 kcal
Fats: 19.3 g
Cholesterol: 88.4 mg
Sodium: 451.9 mg
Carbohydrates: 51.0 g
Dietary Fiber: 7.0 g
Protein: 25.0 g

Mediterranean-Style Eggs with Spinach

Preparation Time: 3 minutes
Cooking Time: 12 minutes **Servings:** 2
Ingredients:

- 2 tablespoons olive oil, melted
- 4 eggs, whisked
- 5 ounces fresh spinach, chopped
- 1 medium-sized tomato, chopped
- 1 teaspoon fresh lemon juice
- ½ teaspoon coarse salt
- ½ teaspoon ground black pepper
- ½ cup of fresh basil, roughly chopped

Directions:

1. Add the olive oil to an Air Fryer baking pan. Make sure to tilt the pan to spread the oil evenly.
2. Simply combine the remaining ingredients—except for the basil leaves—whisk well until everything is well incorporated.
3. Cook in the preheated oven for 8–12 minutes at 280°F. Garnish with fresh basil leaves. Serve.

Nutritional value:
Calories: 274 kcal   Fat: 23.2g Carbs: 5.7g Protein: 13.7g Sugars: 2.6g Fiber: 2.6g

Tabasco Anzac

Preparation Time: 25 minutes
Cooking Time: 3 hours and 45 minutes
Servings: 4
Ingredients:

- 85g porridge oats
- 85g desiccated coconut
- 85g sultanas
- 100g plain flour
- 100g caster sugar
- 100g butter
- 1 tbsp. golden syrup
- 2 tsp. Tabasco
- 2 tbsp. hot water
- 1 tsp. bicarbonate of soda

Directions:

1. Preheat fan assisted oven to 350F.
2. Positioned the oats, raisins, coconut, flour, and sugar in a bowl.
3. Soften the butter in a small pan and stir inside the golden syrup, Tabsco sauce, and water.
4. Add the bicarbonate of soda and mix well.
5. Add the liquid to the bowl and mix well until all the ingredients are combined.
6. Using a dessert spoon, spoon the mixture onto a buttered baking sheet. Leave about 2.5cm in-between each spoonful to allow room for spreading.
7. Bake in batches for 8-10 minutes until golden.
8. Place the cooked biscuits onto a wire rack to cool.

Nutritional value:

Calories: 270 kcal
Fat: 41 g
Protein: 12 g
Cholesterol: 20 mg
Carbohydrates: 20 g
Sodium: 504 mg

Vegan Edamame Quinoa Collard Wraps

Preparation Time: 5 minutes **Cooking Time:** 15 minutes **Servings:** 4
Ingredients:

For the wrap:

- 2–3 Collard leaves
- ¼ cup Grated carrot
- ¼ cup Sliced cucumber
- ¼ Red bell pepper, chopped into thin strips
- ¼ Orange bell pepper, chopped into thin strips
- ⅓ cup Cooked quinoa - ⅓ Shelled defrosted edamame

For the dressing:

- 3 tablespoons Fresh ginger root, peeled and chopped
- 1 cup Cooked chickpeas
- 1 Garlic clove
- 4 tablespoons Rice vinegar
- 2 tablespoons Low sodium tamari or coconut aminos;
- 2 tablespoons Lime juice - ¼ cup Water
- Few pinches chili flakes
- 1 pack Stevia

Directions:

For the dressing, combine all the ingredients and purée in a food processor until smooth. Pour into a small bowl, and set aside. Place the collar leaves on a flat surface, overlapping one another to create a stronger wrap. Take 1 tablespoon of ginger dressing and blend it up with the prepared quinoa. Spoon the prepared quinoa onto the leaves and shape a simple horizontal line at the closest end. Follow with th edamame and remaining veggie fillings. Drizzle around 1 tablespoon of the ginger dressing on top, then fold the cover's sides inwards. Fold the side of the wrap nearest to you over the fillings, the roll the entire wrap away from you to close it up.

Nutritional value:

Calories: 295 Cal Sugar: 3 g Sodium: 200 mg Fat: 13 g

Hummus
Preparation Time: 10 minutes
Cooking Time: 10 minutes
Servings: 32
Ingredients:

- 4 cups cooked garbanzo beans
- 1 cup water
- 1½ tablespoons lemon juice
- 2 teaspoons ground cumin
- 1½ teaspoon ground coriander.
- 1 teaspoon finely chopped garlic
- ½ teaspoon salt
- ¼ teaspoon fresh ground pepper
- Paprika for decorating

Directions:

1. On a food processor, place together the garbanzo beans, lemon juice, water, garlic, salt and pepper and process it until it becomes smooth and creamy.
2. To achieve the desired consistency, add more water.
3. Then spoon out the hummus in a serving bowl
4. Sprinkle your paprika and serve.

Nutritional value:
Protein: 0.7 g
Carbohydrates: 2.5 g
Dietary Fiber: 0.6 g
Sugars: 0 g
Fat: 1.7 g

Conclusion

Lean proteins and good fats are the basis of this cookbook as for a healthy life. With this cookbook you won't no more run out of ideas on what to eat and enjoy because you will be full of delicious and easy to prepare options.

Happy cooking for a healthier life!

CPSIA information can be obtained
at www.ICGtesting.com
Printed in the USA
BVHW010615240221
R11906200001B/R119062PG600778BVX00014B/7